IF SHE DOESN'T DIE SOON I'LL HAVE TO TAKE HER WITH ME.

Confessions of a Dementia Carer

HELEN BROADHURST

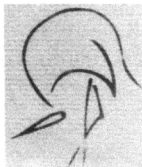

Contents

WHAT IS DEMENTIA?   v

Prologue   1
PART ONE   5
Photos   36
PART TWO   41
Photos   128
PART THREE   137
Photos   168
Afterword   171
Epilogue   175

Acknowledgments   177
CARER SUPPORT   178
AUSTRALIAN RESEARCH FACILITIES   179
SUGGESTED READING   180

WHAT IS DEMENTIA?

DEMENTIA: 'A general loss of cognitive abilities, including impairment of memory as well as one or more of the following: aphasia, apraxia, agnosia, or disturbed planning, organising, and abstract thinking abilities.'

Dementia usually is caused by degeneration in the cerebral cortex, the part of the brain responsible for thoughts, memories, actions, and personality. Death of brain cells in this region leads to the cognitive impairment that characterises dementia.

The most common cause of dementia is Alzheimer's Disease, accounting for half to three-fourths of all cases. The brain becomes clogged with two abnormal structures called neurofibrillary tangles and senile plaques. Neuro-fibrillary tangles are twisted masses of protein fibres inside nerve cells (neurons). Senile plaques are composed of parts of neurons surrounding a group of proteins called beta-amyloid deposits. Why these structures develop is unknown.'

My mother suffered from late onset senile dementia - Alzheimer type.

TO ALL CARERS, EVERYWHERE

'One never goes so far as when one doesn't know where one is going.'
Goethe

Prologue

LATE DECEMBER, 2005

'So, how long will you be staying?'

'Well.' This was tricky. 'I'll be staying on - it's hard to say. I'll be living downstairs ...'

'What? ... You mean 'until I die? Well, I don't know how long that'll be!' My mother leaned forward to peer heavenwards through the window: 'I think He's forgotten me!'

We were sitting on the verandah of her house in Collaroy, Sydney, sharing a cup of tea. I had just arrived after driving my groaning, overloaded little hatchback down from Brisbane to once again take up residence, this time 'for the duration', as I thought of it.

Now I was truly into My Next Project - The Mum Project.

'In the middle of difficulty lies opportunity.'
- Albert Einstein

'Learn by going where you have to go.' - Unknown.

PART ONE

SEPTEMBER, 2004

Widowed at 81, blessed with an iron constitution and robust health, plus a fierce determination to be independent, my mother, Edna Hinder, had managed to remain in her home right through into her nineties.

She had still sewn her own clothes on her vintage treadle Singer and maintained her beloved garden from which, every week, as the self-appointed 'flower lady' of Long Reef Golf Club, she replenished three large display vases in the clubroom. She'd played golf until she turned 90, when she stopped for no reason other than, 'It's ridiculous for someone my age to still be playing.'

As time passed, blessed with a practical wisdom, she sensibly limited car trips to within her own suburb, visiting friends or shopping. Then at 92, when she applied for – and was granted – renewal of her drivers' license, she voluntarily surrendered it and sold her car.

'I'm getting older and DON'T want to be the cause of an accident now.'

Her driving record was without blemish but the family all heaved a sigh of relief, having experienced some pretty hairy trips with her at the wheel in recent years.

Her 95th summer was the last that she went for the daily morning swim down at the nearby beach. Again, this wasn't because she couldn't. Unfortunately her bathers literally fell apart. On a visit earlier in the season I had repaired them as best I could, because nothing would induce her to consider buying a new pair. Anything new was an extravagance. 'I'll never live long enough to wear it out.' End of story.

At about this time I wrote to my children:

'Is it the indomitable spirit or the fierce independence that enables? I still haven't been able to decide what is the source of strength that allows Mum to live alone into her mid-nineties. Is it sheer willpower?'

Born in 1909, the fifth of nine children (six of them brothers) Mum was a product of her time, brought up in a male-dominated world, where her autocratic father reigned supreme. They were a healthy mob; my grandmother reared all the babies born to her and they all reached at least their late eighties.

She was old enough to remember the WW1 armistice parade: 'At nine, I really didn't know what it was all about but I was given a jam-tin full of pebbles to shake and I felt really excited. There was a brass band and soldiers marching and everyone was cheering!'

Her generation had experienced the Great Depression,

then the Second World War, in which three of her brothers and my father served. All returned unwounded.

~

In the early 2000s as Mum moved into her nineties when early signs of dementia were developing, my brother, Richard and I identified that she was coming ever-closer to a time when she would require increasing support.

She would occasionally initiate a chat about one day perhaps needing to move - we even visited a few retirement villages - but her response was always very negative, declaring she couldn't bear to live in such a place and she wasn't going to think about it 'at this stage.' Her over-riding sentiment was that she didn't EVER want to be looked after – by anyone. Her invariable, firm comment was,

'I'm quite capable of looking after myself, as I always have. I manage perfectly well.'

And she had.

We knew staying in her own home was her heart's desire and we regarded it as vitally important to try and achieve that. The problem was that we lived far from her.

Richard and his wife, Soe, lived in Canberra, with full-time jobs. Being single, working as a freelance artist and renting my cottage in Brisbane, I was the one with the flexi-bility in my life to be able to move in with her.

Though I freely admit it wasn't something I really wanted to do, back in 2002, when she was turning 93, I decided to test the waters. I wrote her a tentative letter suggesting I could move down to Sydney 'some time in the future' but the offer was fiercely rejected. She told Richard that I was not the person she'd ever want to have helping her out. Hmmmnn - I wasn't too surprised.

~

The onset of Mum's dementia was quite subtle, noticeable to us but, while she would occasionally acknowledge being forgetful or absent-minded, she had no real insight into the potential impact serious memory loss would have on her personal behaviour or day-to-day living.

For example, once she'd apparently intended to send me a cheque but had neglected to do so. I found out about it when she complained to my brother that she was waiting for me to thank her and was very disappointed in me. What to do? Pretend that I had received a cheque or tell her she hadn't sent it? Or I would hear from someone who had visited her that Mum was very worried because she hadn't heard from me for a long time, yet I was constantly in contact by phone, as well as by regular letter.

At certain times she'd become very defensive at any suggestion she might be 'losing it' so, tippy-toeing (much against my nature!) became a necessity. The situation was further complicated by the fact that, apart from an inherited familial tremor, which mainly affected her hands, neck and lower jaw, she was still physically very strong, with no chronic health conditions to prompt any change in life-style.

At 93 her eyesight had begun to be affected by macular

degeneration and after she turned 94, on one of my trips I had arranged a hearing aid, much to her initial disgust.

'There's really nothing wrong with my ears. All you young people talk too softly and far too fast.'

Despite her physical capabilities I also organised the Constant Companion personal emergency response service, so valuable in the case of a fall. However, by then her short-term memory was increasingly failing and this last was only marginally successful, since I had to explain over the phone, almost weekly, the purpose of the alarm, reminding her that she needed to wear it around her neck at all times at home, even in the garden. I had arranged for two kind neighbours to be the first response.

The vain hope was that it might become a habit. She would agree, then scoff when I explained that it gave me reassurance knowing she could call for help at the press of a button since I lived so far away. The invariable terse retort: 'Good Heavens! I don't need anything; I wouldn't want to bother anyone.'

Fortunately, her vigour didn't diminish and the device never had to be used, because I subsequently discovered that she did get into a habit. She always wore it - when she went out – NEVER AT HOME! It was seen as a 'special necklace', carefully hung on her dressing-table mirror and faithfully draped around her neck before she went shopping.

So, throughout 2003-4, Richard and I had each commuted to her Sydney home as often as we could to check on her, spending long hours in discussion on the phone, about the age-old question: 'What's best for Mum?'

With growing concern for her future well-being, worried about things like fires caused by the stove being left on, or losing the general capacity to look after herself properly, we decided that despite her previous rejection, my moving in was going to be the ultimate solution. But, convincing Mum was quite another- very delicate - matter.

All I could do was keep suggesting, periodically, that I move down to Sydney.

As a freelance place-making community artist, my work took me all over Queensland, doing street and park beautifications as well as school artist-residencies, parades and festivals. I began only taking on short-term projects, not booking myself up too far ahead, always poised to make the move when the time was right.

So it had come as a great relief in August 2004, when, after years of denial of any need for assistance, when I once again suggested, for the umpteenth time that, at this age, to 'have a bit of backup' probably would be a sensible idea, she finally agreed. She had just turned 95.

I wasted no time …

Those lead-up years had allowed me to think through how I could successfully attempt to care for her. My mother and I had had a fairly cordial long-distance relationship for 43 years (since I had married and left to live in P.N.G. aged 20.) Both being quite independent types, we'd never needed to acknowledge that living in too close proximity would almost certainly end in friction.

Over more than four decades, our total time together had probably been less than 12 months.

She had travelled to be with me for the births of my

three children, providing wonderful, wise, practical support and she had made just two short trips to stay with us in the 30 years since we'd returned from P.N.G.

My family had settled in North Queensland in 1975 after Niugini Independence and with three growing children I'd only been able to make short biannual visits over the years. In 1988, when I was 45, my husband and I separated. This meant I was working full-time, with sparse means and limited opportunity for taking breaks. However, more recently, as she'd aged, I'd driven down to Sydney two or three times a year. Despite not being together very often, we always kept close contact, writing weekly letters throughout the entire time and of course, there were regular phone-calls.

My primary objective was to enable her to stay in her own familiar surroundings, maintaining her dignity and sense of independence, keeping her as happy as I could - without her ever becoming aware of my purpose. Her pride was paramount but I also identified the necessity to achieve this while maintaining my own health. I was very aware of the detrimental impact stress can have on the body.

~

Fortunately, throughout my adult years, life had caused me to relocate many times. I had made my home in more than 35 houses.

From age 20, married to a Patrol Officer, whose work often took him out bush for weeks on end, for over 12 years I had lived on somewhat remote out-stations in Niugini. In the early days there was no transport apart from official government vehicles, so no opportunity to leave, no shops or other diversions and very limited social contacts.

Depending on the posting, there might be up to half a dozen other expatriate officers from different government departments, some married, some single.

Living in a very small community in a foreign environment necessitates keeping things cordial without becoming too intimate with anyone. There's no-one to confide in except through the mail, which meant a six week turn around at best. This experience equipped me with lots of practical skills and a fair degree of self-sufficiency.

While there were some difficult times, especially when my husband and I argued, I loved it.

For the past ten years working all over regional Queensland, I had been constantly on the move, often living for months in comparative isolation, as an outsider, in small communities.

So I was very used to relocating, adapting and being self-reliant. My method, when starting a project, after taking up residence in a new community where nothing was familiar, was to identify the constraints, research and discover the available local resources (both human and material) engage with as many people from the community as I could, develop the strategies, then manage.

The boss I had when I was 18 had a favourite instruction: 'Think and Cope'. This became one of my mottos. When presented with a problem I can't immediately resolve, I take it on board by visualising a long, wide beach in my brain. I throw the question onto the beach, set it aside, then mentally imagine the wind and tides moving it around to join up with other flotsam and jetsom. I trust that a solution will emerge in time and it always does; a chance meeting with a complete stranger might bring a different idea - or the necessary skill - or I'll read or hear something that triggers a resolution.

I decided that looking after Mum, although it was a very different circumstance from any I had previously experienced, was simply to be regarded as a project and since project success is essential, I would use my formula to develop the coping strategies to manage this situation. It was up to me.

~

Firstly, I knew we couldn't possibly share her living space. We were both too used to living alone.

After she agreed that I would move to Sydney, knowing she would probably forget our discussion once I returned north and begin to baulk, I followed up by telling her I needed to go down there for a 'small project' and asked if I could take up residence in the unused room under her house, which I knew I could turn into a bed-sit. We discussed this regularly over the next six weeks, while I fulfilled my last commitment out in Quilpie, South West Queensland.

Always very generous, she readily agreed to the arrangement, thinking she was doing me a favour. I did sometimes mention that while I was there I could provide that 'bit of back-up' if she ever needed it but I was very

careful to maintain the concept that it would primarily be
fulfilling my own need.

She was particularly delighted at the prospect of having
my dog, Banjo, around. She absolutely loved dogs but had
denied herself the pleasure of owning one since her last dog
died, some 12 years before. This was because it might
outlive her and this (apparently) wouldn't be fair to the
animal. Again no amount of persuasion or assurance that
I'd take the dog if necessary had made any difference.

In addition, my car would be a plus because she was
increasingly finding shopping trips in the community bus
quite stressful. She had become disorientated in the supermarket on more than one occasion, delaying the other
elderly passengers and causing herself great embar-
rassment.

In vain, both Richard and I had tried to organise a taxi
for weekly shopping trips but this was firmly rejected - in
her limited experience a taxi was a luxury beyond compre-
hension.

Seven weeks later I had wound up all my affairs in
Queensland, sub-let my cottage and moved to Sydney. By
keeping in close contact about the plans, I was confident
she expected me but I was dismayed to discover on arrival
that, being the consummate generous hostess, she had
singlehandedly moved all her clothes and personal items
out of the master bedroom down into the, at that stage,
rather derelict room under the house.

My protestations that I definitely would not take over
her room were swept aside. I moved my cases into her

spare room and carted boxes of the household items I'd brought downstairs.

'You can stay down there for now if you choose, but tomorrow I plan to start washing walls and painting. I've got my portable stove and a microwave so I'll be able to set up a kitchenette and in about two weeks I expect to move in.' I knew I needed to be very firm.

I didn't want a confrontation at that crucial stage so I made light of it all and took advantage of the novelty of my arrival, by taking her with me on shopping expeditions.

Her bedroom remained empty for several nights as she resolutely took herself downstairs every evening, picking her way among the drop-cloths, paint pots and trestles until eventually she quietly began bringing her clothes back upstairs.

Over the next couple of months, with many sorties to nearby op-shops, acquiring bits of furniture and various other treasures, I proceeded to convert the downstairs room into a delightful, completely independent living space, setting up a cooking area and re-vamping the primitive bathroom.

We quietly established our new relationship. Mum took a great interest in all my activities; seeing me busy pleased her and provided diversion.

At that stage, she required minimal care, so my days were full of restoring furniture, making blinds, tiling the bathroom and painting - nest building.

I also set up a little office for myself in the small, hardly-used third bedroom upstairs, where I could work at my computer and be within earshot without seeming to be in her space.

Of course, I had no way of knowing what the future held. I learned long ago not to have expectations about anything but rather, to deal with whatever life throws up. I certainly didn't envisage dramas such as involvement with the police, or the spectacular accidents Mum managed to create.

That was all ahead.

~

Having experienced excellent health for her entire life and being a passionate gardener she had always maintained regular physical activity. At 95 she could still comfortably squat or sit down on the ground, weeding, for hours on end, then stand up without using support. She was insulted by offers of assistance when walking, pushing any prof-fered helping hand away, even when negotiating a kerb or rough ground. In fact at that stage, I had trouble keeping up with her.

Have I mentioned? She was stubborn!

So the caring needs were quite minimal to begin with. I made sure the stove wasn't left on, assisted with shopping and did occasional housework (although she regarded this as interference so I had to wait until she was down in the garden or napping in her chair to get in a bit of vacuuming.) To clean the bathroom, I pretended to be using the toilet with the door closed.

Mum wasn't a particularly fussy housekeeper - her

garden took precedence. However, she always had vases of flowers throughout, arranging them herself. In fact one large wall vase necessitated standing on a low stool to arrange the flowers. I learned to bite my tongue re suggesting the possibility of a fall. There was no question of either letting me fill it or relocating the vase - it was a fixture and being left empty wasn't remotely an option, so quite early on I developed my most scientific of strategies – crossing my fingers!

Despite gradually losing the capacity to weigh the ingredients and requiring increasing assistance with the oven, Mum also never forgot about making her shortbread from the recipe she'd used when I was a child. The rusty old balance scales would be dragged out of the cupboard, a 500g pat of butter produced (to be cut up as substitute for the long-lost weights) and she'd find me wherever I was. 'I need to make biscuits.'

My job was to prompt the recipe: I'd start, 'Half a pound …' and she'd join in with a sing-song chant: 'of flour! Half a pound of butter and a quarter of a pound of castor sugar.' Then she'd add triumphantly, 'And a pinch of salt!'

After I weighed and combined the ingredients in the big old bowl she'd take up her position at her aged marble slab, a 'must' for every kitchen. I was invariably informed that biscuits HAD to be kneaded on a marble slab and she'd happily work away at the dough, pressing, scraping and balling the mixture until it was just right.

Another 'must' was the correct preparation of the oven. Two multi-layered newspaper strips had to be placed on the oven shelf under the biscuit pan - a reversion to the old days of primitive fuel stoves, which lacked thermometers. When I first arrived, charred remnants of paper littering the oven floor from many previous batches fluttered out every time it was opened - an early cleaning job.

Biscuit-making sometimes happened two or three times a week – or perhaps she wouldn't think of it for a period - so it did tend to be feast or famine, although she never quite ran out and always had some to offer visitors. It was jolly good shortbread too.

She tended to wear clothes well past their washing time (not to mention their use-by date!) Many of her clothes were pretty tatty. Based on the swimming costume reasoning, she wouldn't buy anything new. For years, she had used the same pattern to make herself many loose overblouses, her customary summer-wear over slacks.

Unfortunately, the tremor caused her to spill food and despite draping a large cloth over herself when eating, food stains adorned everything. If we were going shopping and I gently pointed out that quite a bit of her meal had dribbled down her front, hoping she'd take this as a prompt to change, quick as a flash she'd whip it over her head and reverse it. After all, the back was perfectly clean! I knew better than to actually suggest a replacement.

All in all I got pretty nifty at sleight of hand, whipping dirty clothes into the washing machine before she put them on again or if I got caught in her room when collecting, I'd explain that I only had a half-load and she'd be doing me a favour if I added a few of her half- dirty garments.

I became adept at overseeing food preparation without

her knowledge and generally ducking and diving around every activity - helping without helping.

I knew contentment was being in control of her own life. My job was to keep her content.

In dealing with Mum's dementia I rapidly learned I could resist or yield – there's always a choice. When I resisted the consequences were dire.

She had a strong personality and didn't know when she was being irrational or difficult. If she perceived that I was crowding her or trying to make her do something she didn't want to do, she could fly off the handle very quickly.

'You treat me worse than your dog! Go away!'

I'd remove myself but she'd hang onto her resentment and I'd receive the silent treatment, which she was very good at. In the early months she could maintain coldness for a day or more.

~

Complications threatened when she took it into her head every now and again to walk down to the pharmacy several blocks away. Once decided, she'd be off, shopping bag looped over her shoulder.

Apart from eye vitamins and drops her only regular medication was half a sleeping tablet nightly, an established habit due to always being a light sleeper. I suspected that their efficacy had long passed but old habits don't. Having repeat prescriptions safely lodged at the pharmacy, she tended to trot off to get a refill well before it was required. I'd discovered quite a cache of tablets in a drawer after I moved in. I had to dismiss the brief thoughts about this being intentional. I removed the excess packets and if Mum noticed I never heard about it.

To me these excursions were a sign of a sub-conscious need to prove self-sufficiency. Offers to drive her were always refused - she really did like to walk.

My only course of action was for Banjo to have yet another impromptu outing so I could follow her at a discreet distance. She usually managed the first leg success-fully, following her established route from the house with me shadowing her. Even if she'd looked back I doubt that she'd have recognised me but I stayed across the road and hid behind trees when necessary. On the return journey, though, just one deviation when she left the store would send her off-track.

Loitering across the road, I'd watch her blithely take off in the wrong direction. This was when I'd duck around the block and 'meet' her. 'Oh! Hullo! What a nice surprise! I'm just on my way home with Banjo. Let's go together.'

With her abundant energy, the extra distance never bothered her in the least. You could call it 'Care by Stealth.'

Two things she always really enjoyed. I set her hair weekly and I 'visited' - simply spending time sitting with her on her verandah, providing companionship. She, however, always insisted on making the tea since I was the guest.

Her brain had certain fixations, which were re-hashed almost daily, such as whether I was 'comfortable' - a euphemism for well-off - how long she would be able to stay in her home, plus various musings about neighbours or relatives. A major preoccupation was what she had in the bank and concern about whether she had enough money to stay living in her house. Almost daily I'd produce her bankbook, point out the healthy bottom line and write the figure down in large letters, explaining that her aged pension would continue for life, no matter how long she lived. Every day there was the same reaction - amazement. This was reassuring news no-one had ever explained before.

I had to condition myself to accept these dreary repetitions. The challenge was to move to another subject as quickly as possible. She had always been a worrier, imagining dire situations where none existed - an entrenched behaviour. She had no memory of previous, identical discussions and so trying to dismiss a worry with reassurance was useless.

She didn't discriminate re her audience, either. These subjects were brought up with anyone who happened to arrive, including tradesmen. Once, she even bailed up a cold caller, who'd come to the door when I was downstairs. The poor woman was trying to escape when I turned up.

Unfortunately this was somewhat off-putting for her neighbours, who stopped dropping by once I moved in and, sadly, it's not usual to have too many contemporaries once you reach your nineties. Mum had seen off all her old friends.

A week after moving in I took her to the funeral of a very old friend, Peggy, who she had known since the war years, when both their husbands were away. She created a diversion when, while walking between the chapel and the reception room her half slip ever-so-slowly slid down from under her skirt! Quite unconcerned, she blithely stepped out of it, laughing, and continued walking, leaving me to hastily stuff it into my bag. It briefly lightened the mood and drew a wry comment from Peggy's daughter, Sandra:

'Trust Edna to upstage Mum!'

I spent some time secretly repairing clothes that were really way past decency.

～

To preserve my patience - and sanity - I very early learned that I must accept her reality and treat each repeated experience as if it was the first time, just as she herself believed. The key was to switch off – to detach - concentrate on saying something to satisfy her then try to divert her onto another subject.

Contradiction or pointing out that we'd already had this discussion disturbed her and caused more grief than it was worth. She'd become agitated, distressed, very disoriented and angry. She'd accuse me of lying or trying to upset her if I tried to correct a story or fact. It was as if her mind could briefly glimpse the gaps and disconnections; as if she subconsciously comprehended a failure and was striving to register full cognition - to 'connect the dots'.

I have since read about explicit and implicit memory, explicit being conscious memories that can be recalled - often very old ones - and implicit being more unconscious - the skill of cleaning one's teeth or other regular daily tasks without actually thinking about them. I am eternally grateful that Mum's implicit memory remained relatively intact throughout. She voluntarily bathed, cleaned teeth, etc. without prompting but her explicit memory was far more fragmented.

Apparently the blood-brain barrier is involved. At the time of writing there have been experiments on mice, where ultrasound waves applied to an affected brain can briefly open the blood-brain barrier and the subject reverts to much greater cognisance.

I wonder if this can occur spontaneously because sometimes Mum would surprise me by her sharp responses.

To some degree I think I have a natural capacity for detachment. Or perhaps those experiences in P.N.G. and working in small communities where I learned to avoid gossip and stay focussed contributed to this. I found I could switch off and not indulge in an emotional reaction.

I treated her as an important elderly person, who I needed to respect and keep happy, no matter what, rather than my mother being irritating. This detachment was an attribute for which I became extremely grateful - especially after Mum ceased to know who I was.

While I learned never to remind her about anything that had occurred recently, typically, the old memories were always accessible.

I'd encourage her to tell me about being the first girl in her hometown, Dubbo, to wear slacks, which she made herself after seeing a photo in a magazine. Back in the nineteen twenties this was very daring! And the highlight of her life – a cruise to Fiji from Sydney.

It was the Great Depression; Mum had always worked as her father's secretary - not necessarily what she wanted -

but her oldest sister was the designated 'stay-at-home with Mother' daughter and the middle one had married at 18. My stern, autocratic grandfather needed a secretary and Mum had done a typing course so her job fate was sealed.

Marriage was every girl's ultimate dream and my parents became engaged in their early twenties but Mum very boldly decided she wanted to have one overseas adventure before settling down. So she saved during their seven year engagement and planned a cruise from Sydney to Fiji - alone.

It should be remembered that in those days organising a trip from a country town entailed writing several letters over a considerable period of time; this was before long-distance phone-calls and, of course, travel agents didn't exist.

She didn't tell her father until she'd actually bought both the boat and train tickets, presenting the venture as a fait accompli. Despite his disapproval of such an outlandish venture, my grandfather's only option was to give his bless-ing, since there was no question of getting a refund. And, amazingly, on the eve of departure he gave her a signed, blank cheque - to be used only in an emergency.

'There was even an article about my cruise in the local paper when I got home!' In those days, in a small country town, any overseas trip was seriously exotic!

The best memory - her eyes would light up with glee at the thought. 'I saw a beautiful set of silk underwear in the shop on board. It was very expensive - I really felt I shouldn't buy it - but it was too lovely. I got up my nerve and used Dad's cheque!'

After all, she was an engaged girl and this would be a truly special addition to her Glory Box (the traditional collection of linen and special items in preparation for marriage, customary in those times.) Not only did she wear it for her own wedding but she also loaned the set to her best friend, Elma, when she married Mum's brother, my Uncle Bill.

Another regular story was the one about when the maypole fell on her head. She'd lean forward and make me feel the scar.

'I was only little - maybe in second class - and I was very shy, but we used to do maypole dancing. I was trying to do all the steps, winding in and out with the other kids. Then suddenly the pole fell over right on top of me! It cracked my head! I do remember that. I was terribly embarrassed because the teacher - I can't remember her name but she was really nice - had to pull all the ribbons away and lift up the pole and everyone was watching.'

'It was bleeding and she put a handkerchief onto it and took me down to the chemist. He patched it up properly and the teacher took me home to Mum. But! Do you know what he gave me - the chemist? A banana! I'd never, ever seen one before! I'd only seen a picture in one of the schoolbooks! I took it home and Mum made me give half to my little brother but I can still remember how it tasted - so sweet!'

Telling those and many other familiar tales kept her happy. Many hours we sat chatting on Mum's verandah with our tea, Banjo lying nearby.

~

Initially it shocked me to realise how devious I was becoming - prevaricating, avoiding direct responses, trotting out whatever version of a story I felt she expected, developing the capacity to look her in the eye and tell a complete untruth.

However, I knew that her equilibrium was the most important factor so we would wend our way through conversations, with me improvising and keeping my fingers crossed that she didn't retain any details, because I wasn't confident that I could keep my own stories straight!

I always strived to protect her from the distress and agitation that could flare up so rapidly when that 'fog' suddenly cleared and the cognitive processes would allow her brain to register that the mind connections weren't quite functioning.

I sensed that the subconscious striving was always somewhere there, just below the surface. In addition, her anger was definitely worth avoiding!

A lot of the time our interactions were really funny, even though the fact that I was her daughter would sometimes drift away.

A typical exchange: the weekly hair-setting session, where she'd be on a stool in front of the long mirror set into her familiar old art deco dressing table, with the two sets of drawers on each side, their tops cluttered with rollers and pins. Mum still had most of the furniture they'd bought when they first married. I don't think it had ever occurred to her to buy new furniture.

I was winding rollers into her hair. Almost done.

'Are you a hairdresser?'

'No.'

Long pause, 'I had a daughter who was.'

'Did you really?'

It was true. 48 years before, when I was 17 I had left a hairdressing apprenticeship after two years, due to developing dermatitis. Here was another old memory, quite intact.

She passed me another roller. Looked at my reflection in the mirror. 'Yes - Helen - That's my daughter's name.'

Wondering where this conversation might go I asked:

'Where's Helen now?'

'Oh! ... She lives ... somewhere else.' The eyes started wandering. Cue - change of subject.

Another time: I'd poured her tea into her favourite cup.

'Who are you married to now?' These questions came apropos nothing.

'I'm not married. I haven't been married for nearly twenty years.'

Pause ... 'Aaah!' ... then, looking at me quizzically:

'Who were you married to?'

'Peter'

'Oh?' ... sip of tea, 'Peter who?'

'Broadhurst – that is my name now.'

'Oh ... Peter Broadhurst!' An even longer pause, then (query in the voice) 'Helen! ... Helen married him.'

'Er, yes, that's right.'

After another slow sip of tea: 'So, do you know if Helen is still married to him?'

'Uh? No, she's not. They're divorced.'

I was saved from having to extricate myself from this one because the word 'divorce' was a hook for a practiced opinion, delivered with confident satisfaction.

'Yes, that's what people do nowadays. My mother and your mother stayed married. The world is a very different place now.'

At times I had a surreal feeling of having fallen down the rabbit-hole with the Mad Hatter just around the next corner!

In her mind she was sitting on her verandah drinking tea with a guest, so 'hostess mode' had kicked in. It always amazed me that she could hide the fact that she didn't have a clue who she was talking to. It seemed innate. A good hostess will offer more tea and never embarrass a guest - a guest must be catered for in every way. She never lost the knack of using certain polite sentences that suited multiple social situations, including assuring people that she remembered who they were, without ever actually saying a name.

This isn't uncommon. Many full-time carers despair, when family members occasionally visit and are convinced that 'Auntie, or 'Granma' knows them. They protest that she isn't nearly as bad as the poor carer has described.

Only other carers know.

Living separately, ultimately, proved to be the key to success I believe, because, to the end, despite increasing irrationality, delusions and extreme memory loss, at those times when Mum's distress became overwhelming and we'd suddenly be in a scene with her shouting at me, accusing me of lying or trying to upset her (almost always because I had mismanaged) telling her I was going back to my place would defuse the situation. That ingrained sense of the right to individual privacy remained and she almost always respected my space.

Many a time, seething, I retreated downstairs when a situation became too difficult. It was either that, or if I had to get right out of the way, I'd announce an urgent need to walk Banjo, which I knew she would approve of.

Timing was crucial.

~

Mum had always been an avid reader of the *Sydney Morning Herald*, delivered daily, as well as books from the library but gradually, this became more and more difficult. One of her constantly-stated regrets was that she 'couldn't read any more.'

Both her eye doctor and I had patiently explained to her many times over the years that macular degeneration couldn't be assisted by stronger glasses but she never stopped asking me to take her back for another test. I obtained a book-reading magnifier from the Blind Society and strengthened her reading lamp but nothing seemed to help. Eventually Mum agreed for the paper delivery to be reduced to Saturdays only and she valiantly worked at reading it day after day.

I think it was as much that her concentration was affected as the eyesight, because she was religious in applying her eye-drops and regular tests indicated there was no measurable further deterioration.

Also, she always collected the mail, managing to distinguish which letters were hers, which mine and she could spot any tiny piece of fluff on the carpet, which she'd bend down and retrieve.

Mum truly mourned the loss of reading, something she mentioned often. It made me very sad. I tried borrowing audio books from the library but again, she seemed unable to follow the story and in any case the previous day's chapter would fly off into the ether so there could be no continuity, just another cause for frustration.

～

At the end of 2004, about three months after I took up residence, my daughter Kriket and her partner, Mark, suggested that they would like a spell living in Sydney while Mark finished writing his PHD thesis so they offered to take on the caring duties. The 'short spell' extended to 12 months.

And so, after Christmas, when Richard and Soe had spent a few days with Mum while Banjo and I drove back to Brisbane, the reins were handed over to Kriket and Mark, who moved into my little bed-sit downstairs with their dog, Modj.

Mum accepted this change with little comment. As far as she understood, they needed a place to live in Sydney and she was happy to have them there. 'Modj' was soon christened 'Podge' and from then on, every dog she saw was called 'Podge', including Banjo.

An email came from Kriket in Feb 2005:

'I had a couple of good talks to Nan the last couple of days re you and your work and the fact that you probably won't be back down here for a few months - middle of the year or so. She seemed O.K. - said she wondered if you needed to work or wanted to work. I asked her if she would prefer you to be down here with her and she thought about it for a bit and then said it is not up to her - so I asked her if it was what she wanted, regardless - she said she had not really thought about it. She seems confused more than anything at WHY we would want to stay in Sydney but happy for us to be down here (SHE is O.K! doesn't need anyone here.)

But after a bit she opened up and I told her that if she wanted to do anything in particular or go to any places we could take her. She said she is happy working in the garden but some days finds it a bit much after gardening all week.

I said well that's natural to get a bit tired of the same old, same old and we could go off somewhere on some days - she said yes she would be interested in going to plant nurseries etc. (but not sight-seeing) so I will endeavour to coax her out.

She LOVED going to DJ's last week - looked at all the 'garments' and checked out how they were made.'

As time passed she became more and more unpredictable.

In April, another email came from Krik:

'We didn't hear the phone last night when you rang but there was a break-through! Nan came downstairs calling out 'Kriket, Kriket, Helen is on the phone'. This is the first time she has ever called me by that name!!!!!! Felt quite weird.'

Always avoiding nicknames, a stickler for never shortening anyone's name, Mum was the only person who called Kriket by her correct name, 'Celia' and was still remembering it at that stage, though by the end of the year, when she still remembered 'Mark', Kriket had become 'her'.

She deteriorated noticeably throughout 2005 becoming disturbed and muddled more often, not recognising well-known people and increasingly preferring to be home, happy to work in her garden and to sit and try to read.

Despite all efforts, at times she became suspicious of Kriket and Mark's presence and sometimes she was down-right hostile, especially mid-year, when Kriket and Mark planned to go to New Zealand for a fortnight and I was to take over.

During those early months, it was still difficult to gauge how much to tell Mum when anything was planned. The tippy-toeing about why we were there had to be maintained.

We planned it so that they would tell her just a few days before their departure with me ready to follow up on the phone, saying I was coming for a visit and would be minding Modj.

However Mum happened to be in a perceptive phase and became very angry.

'I'm perfectly capable of looking after Podge. I've had dogs all my life. Do you think I don't know what to do?'

'Well, no, of course you do. But she needs to have a couple of walks a day and you mightn't feel like doing that. Besides, I want to come and visit you.' I tried to placate her.

'Rubbish! You don't trust me! You think I'm a useless old woman and I can't be on my own. Why don't you all just go away? I don't want anyone here.'

Such situations could lead to a prolonged period of

disgruntlement with her agonising about being a burden, followed by great agitation, which led to tight-lipped non-co-operation so Krik and Mark had a few hairy days.

By the time I arrived she had settled down again to some degree and Krik and Mark had their holiday.

They managed to lead a fairly normal life, admirably supporting Mum but I remember one occasion when I had a very tearful Krik on the phone.

Richard and Soe were coming to visit for a few days and, after helping Mum to prepare their room and making sure the fridge was stocked etc., Kriket and Mark planned to go off for a break themselves.

They were in the car ready to drive away when suddenly Mum was out at the kerb banging on the window, imperiously ordering them to stop. Krik wound the window down.

'Don't go yet. The beds aren't right. They have to be pushed together to make a double bed.'

'The beds are always kept separate. That's how Soe and Richard always have them,' Krik assured her. 'I've left them exactly the way they have been for years.'

Mum angrily brushed this aside as she began tugging at the car door handle. Krik could see this escalating out of control so she stayed in the car. Both she and Mark had been working hard all morning and they were very keen to get away by themselves.

'This is my house. I know what Richard and Soe want. I want you to come back and rearrange the beds.'

Knowing that this would only make difficulties for them as Richard suffers from a debilitating muscle-wasting disease, necessitating a wheelchair and beginning to run late, Krik decided that retreat was the only option.

'We have to go now, Nana. We're running late. Honestly, everything is organised. It'll be O.K.'

Mark began slowly driving down the road. The parting shout from an irate five-foot-nothing grandmother, standing in the middle of the road: 'Go to Hell!' was decidedly disturbing for poor Krik, since Mum's most extreme expletive was usually 'darn'.

I was always available to take over if it became too onerous but they managed wonderfully 'til the end of the year, when Mark finished his thesis. Richard and Soe stepped in again while they headed back north to celebrate Christmas with me.

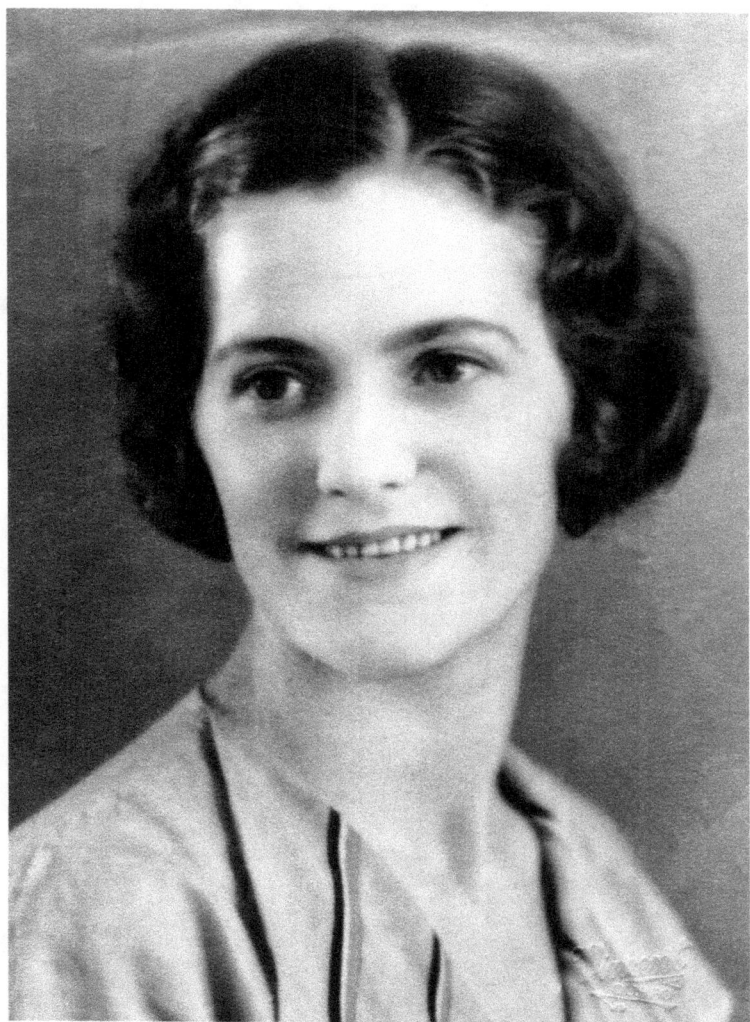

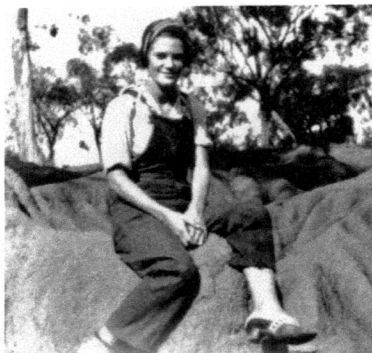

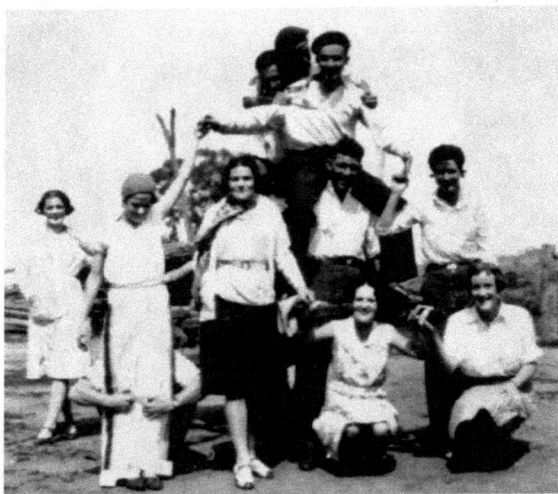

The trend setter - the only girl not in a skirt. Over page: On Board the Strathnavor - cruise to Fiji. Last page: Honeymoon golf.

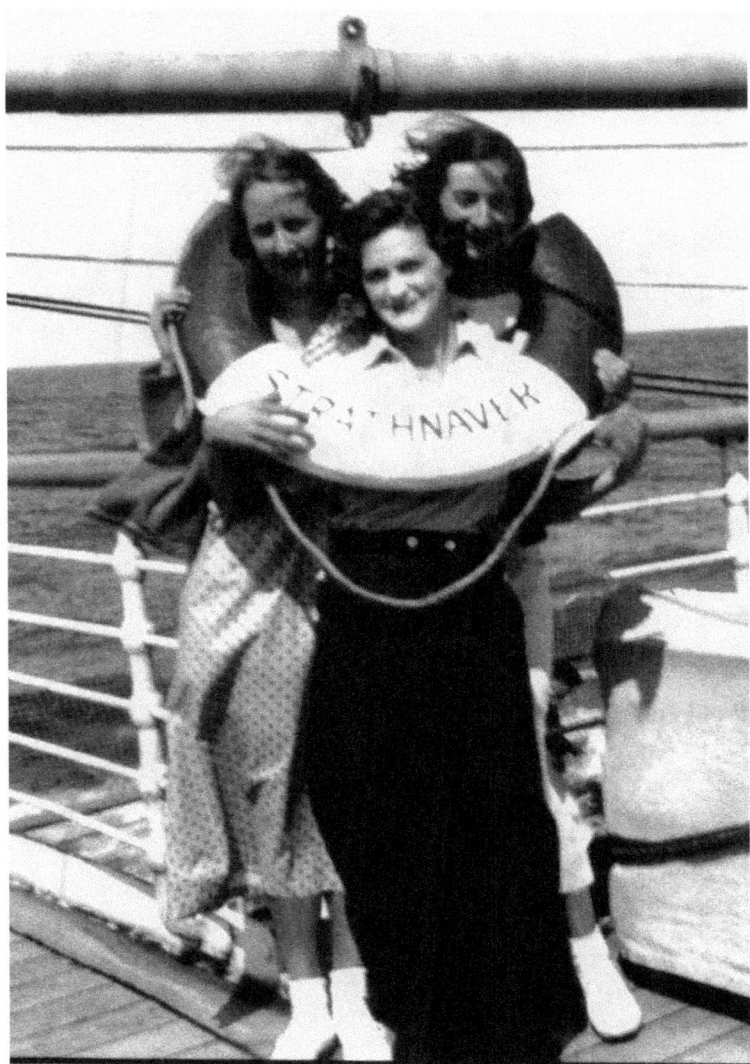

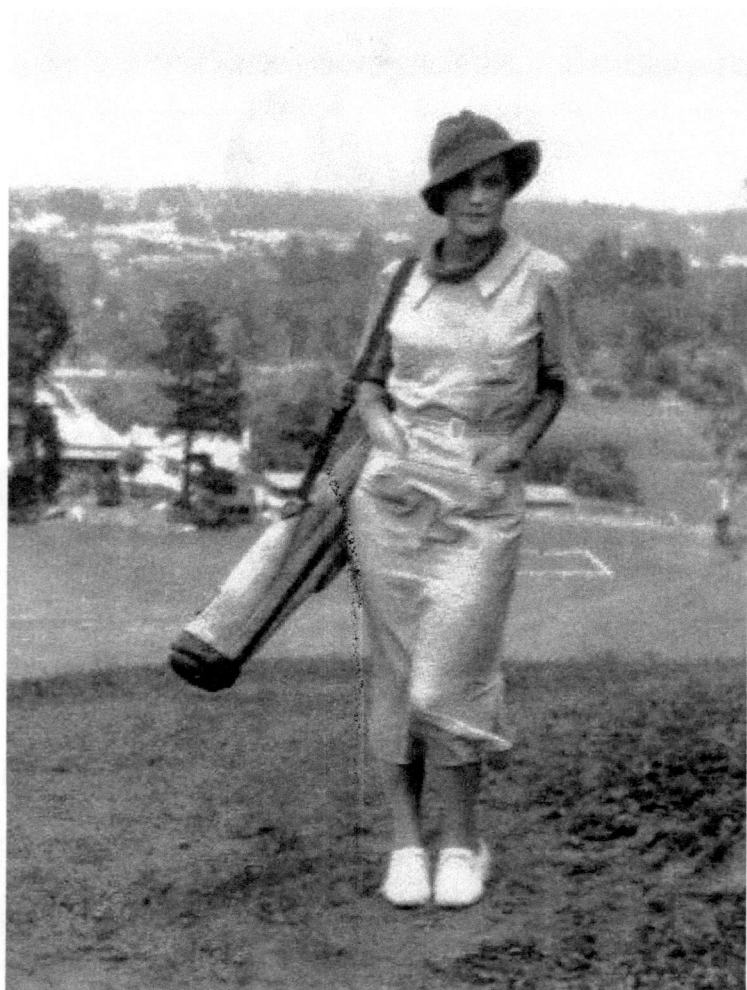

Learn to accept those things you cannot alter,
not blindly, but with full understanding.
- unknown.

PART TWO

So – late December 2005 - there we were back out on Mum's verandah together. On that day, from her point of view, she'd simply had a succession of visitors. Kriket and Mark had left as Richard and Soe arrived before Christmas and I turned up the day they departed so she saw me as just another visitor. At that stage she still knew who I was.

My mother's dementia always kept every experience new and fresh. For 16 months she'd constantly had family members living with her and although at times she'd perceived that someone was 'hovering', she didn't recall how continuous it had been.

Now she was asking how long I'd be staying.

It was always impossible to predict just where her mind was 'at' – it could be so mercurial – and I hadn't seen her for several months. But, aware that she still strongly resisted the idea of 'being looked after' and not knowing how she was coping with all the changes, the last thing I was going to discuss was what was actually happening.

I had previously experienced that cold, abusive wrath, which could be maintained for extended periods. She still had the quick temper and if she felt wronged, she could contain a cold hostility, refusing to communicate with whoever had upset her.

I was determined to start off on the right foot.

The project was to keep her happy by living in her own familiar surroundings for as long as I reasonably could. However, I had no illusions. Experience had taught me the debilitating impact stress can have on one's health. At 45 the effects of prolonged conflict toward the end of my marriage had briefly driven me onto tranquilisers, and at 63 I had no intention of repeating this. I promised the family I would do my best, but I was not prepared to lose my own health through caring.

My one proviso was I was not a martyr. If I decided I couldn't cope, we would need to organise a Plan B.

Mum was 96 and a half. It might be imagined that this caring situation would not be for such a very long time but I had no illusions about that either; while the brain was deteriorating, the body most definitely was not!

How to describe my Mum? Her conditioning was to be dutiful, hard-working, frugal, 'sensible' and stoic. She set – and lived by – high standards - the Protestant Work Ethic personified. She expected no less from her children. My grandfather, Mum's Dad, had been an elder in the Anglican church - a pillar of the community - and she had told me many times that throughout her childhood, as the jostled, middle child of a tribe of kids, she had been afraid of him. The church was involved in separating Aboriginal children from their families under the draconian, early 20th century laws and the family knew their father was on the committee.

'I was always terrified if I got into trouble that I'd be sent away like them.'

Very capable, supremely practical and creative, 'do-it-yourself' was the only way she knew; she sewed almost all her own clothes and had taught herself upholstery, re-covering all her furniture over the years, as well as that of many friends and relatives.

She loved colour - especially the peacock colours. Three of her wingback lounge chairs were deep teal and the fourth was royal purple. A vintage lounge was covered in a brightly patterned linen incorporating these colours plus all the others to be found in a peacock's plumage. Her dresses and tops all echoed this.

In her fifties she even went to a night-class to learn how to build the new bathroom cabinets she wanted, installing them herself.

Sadly, she never could manage to accept praise for herself, always playing down her achievements, becoming crushingly embarrassed at any attention.

My mother never reached her full potential. She was born at the wrong time, when strict, traditional family structures were firmly entrenched. Being a good wife and mother dominated her life and she mostly suppressed all other inclinations. I've often imagined how she'd have blos-somed if she'd been born 50 years later.

She viewed men with a somewhat jaundiced eye (though doctors could do no wrong) and loved children and animals. She would volunteer to help anyone in need. She was an extremely kind person yet toward her family she was very judgemental.

Mum also had an unfortunate capacity for holding a grudge. Two of my cousins had been 'wiped' long ago after offending her. I recall one was because my cousin, who worked in an allied health field, 'interfered' and dared to question some medical treatment Mum was undergoing, making an alternative suggestion. I have no idea why that was enough to decide she wanted nothing more to do with her niece. I wasn't involved, living far away, but I had suffered my share of periods of silence over the years, because I'd perhaps written something in a letter that disappointed her. I'd notice a succession of weekly letters came only from my father, whereas they usually took it in turns to write. These situations were only defused when I proffered the olive branch.

At the same time she was wise and tolerant in many ways. As children we were taught never to display discrimination in any form and her strong tenets of duty and self-discipline were also passed on to Richard and me.

In 1952, when I was ten, we relocated to a two-storey house in Sydney, large enough to accommodate Mum's ageing parents, who lived with us for the next decade.

In many ways, I believe her entrenched habits of life, including her stubbornness and a strong sense of right and wrong, combined with an excellent gene pool, contributed to her longevity. She had never altered her lifelong, traditional healthy eating patterns - grapefruit and cereal for breakfast, salad lunches followed by fruit, then meat and at least three veg. dinners, also followed by fruit - plus 8 glasses of water a day, beginning with three upon waking.

She took 'having a proper meal' to extremes and had inculcated this into me to the extent that I remember being in my thirties before finally convincing myself that I didn't need to feel guilty for occasionally giving my kids a meat pie for dinner!

I believe she suffered all her life from a severe inferiority complex. This was expressed in a number of ways, more particularly in the fact that it prevented her from ever being able to truly acknowledge any success by Richard or myself. She couldn't believe that any child she produced would be capable of achieving much at all. She would congratulate us on any achievement, showing pleased interest but there was always a reserve. As children we'd never been encouraged to put ourselves forward in any way.

Possibly because my grandparents were in our house, traditional rules applied. During the fifties, the Australian society I spent my teenage years in was parochial and conservative. I always felt loved but my training was to be dutiful and not question. I definitely had to sit up straight at the table. Richard and I were taught to never go back on our word.

I challenged my grandfather - we clashed - which no doubt caused problems. I don't think he'd ever been confronted by any female in his 80 plus years. But I didn't overtly rebel. I had great respect for my parents and always made decisions considering how they might affect Mum and Dad.

I was into my thirties before I realised that I was never going to impress my mother – would always fall short in some way. It was at this same time, when I finally gave myself permission to relax some of her standards, that meat pies occasionally began appearing on my family dinner table.

This inability to praise me had been demonstrated on my visits over recent years, when I showed her photographs (the physical evidence) of quite major public art projects that I had managed and executed. She clearly couldn't quite believe it. Her invariable comment was to the effect that she didn't understand how I could be working as an artist, 'because you were never any good at art in school.' This is true. I was never a mark-maker - a painter - but, like her, I am creative in other ways. She couldn't accept this.

Similarly, when Richard graduated with his education degree, Dad travelled to Canberra for the ceremony but Mum didn't. Somehow, being there would have forced her to acknowledge her son's achievement.

When I moved in with her for that last stretch I knew that my job was to accept the way she had always been and enable whatever she required without trying to change it - simply to maintain her patterns and try to keep her happy.

Although she would go out of her way to help almost anyone, looking back through my life, I had long since given up trying to do anything for her. For example, long before, when visiting my parents with my family, we would sit down for the evening meal, which she invariably insisted on cooking, then, before the rest of us had finished she'd be out in the kitchen washing up. No amount of protesting, offers to do it later or to 'please leave it' had any effect.

Likewise, our washing would be off the line almost before it had dried. She sometimes carried self-sacrifice and martyrdom to extremes. I could never get a step ahead of her and eventually I had learned to accept that this was simply how she was.

Kind and generous, she had been the Aunt who took people in. Different cousins in need had found a home with my parents for varying extended periods. She was always ready to help someone out but gave no-one, including close friends, a chance to do anything for her. As I've mentioned, she was extremely stubborn and very proud. My mild-mannered, conservative father accommodated her decisions without complaint. A cousin, who lived with us during my late teens, recently told me my Dad was the nicest man she had ever met.

~

Now she was happy to heat up a frozen T.V. dinner at night, always preparing fresh vegetables to eat with it. These would be carefully placed in a metal steamer basket inside a big saucepan with two side handles with just a small amount of water. She earnestly explained, almost nightly, that steaming was the best. The problem was, she also 'knew' it took 20 minutes to cook vegetables.

She was blithely unaware that her ancient saucepan had virtually burned through and I didn't bother to suggest replacing it. My strategy was to regularly scout the op-shops and pick up replicas as spares, which I could substitute each time the current one was burnt beyond retrieval. Lunch was generally a cold salad, so that was safe.

Therefore, with a small amount of tweaking, I allowed her to prepare her own meals as she always had. A couple of times a week I would invite her down to dinner at my place and she loved that – thought of it as a treat.

Every week, she'd exclaim, 'A baked dinner – I haven't had a baked dinner for years!'

Stability and routine were the keys to keeping things on an even keel. Respond and facilitate (plus crossed fingers) were the management tools. By trial and error I learned the strategies to manage and as Mum's mind descended into greater and greater confusion, maintaining the routine increasingly became my most essential tactic.

Fortunately, over time, the dementia did mellow her to some degree.

Most of the time she knew who I was in the early months but occasionally we'd have those interesting conversations about me in the third person. I finally learned not to tell her who I was if she asked. I never forgot that last time when I did:

'Helen'

'Helen who?'

'Helen, … your daughter.'

She stared at me, doubting; I could see the confusion, the dawning realisation. Then came the stricken reply: 'How could I forget my own daughter?'

Over time I met other carers who anguished over this

lack of recognition by their loved one but I accepted it as a simple fact. I saw absolutely no point in agonising over the fact that my mother didn't know me - it wasn't personal. This was another situation where detachment became very useful. Besides, since visitors weren't subjected to the same judgmental scrutiny as family, becoming incognito - the friendly person who lived downstairs - automatically made my life much easier - a definite plus!

~

Mislaying everything is also an inevitable symptom of dementia. Kriket had suffered the frustration of having to organise Mum's hearing aid to be replaced four times in six months.

Mum wore the free, standard issue, small 'inside-the-ear' type which requires a little bit of manipulation to extricate by a tiny wisp of flexible tubing. She would insist on keeping the hearing aid in until she went to bed, when she would remove it, along with her bottom teeth. (For some reason she never removed the top denture at night.)

Needless-to-say they would be left in various secret places in the house, rarely together, which meant a search almost every morning. Sometimes we could be lucky but she would often have to go without either, or both, for days, which meant having the T.V. at the highest volume and all conversation several decibels up. I remember an occasion when, after such a period, I found the denture, broken in two, down in the garden. On investigating the windowsill above I discovered the little cloth bag that she sometimes put them in tangled in the vine there. She'd oh-so-carefully popped the teeth into the bag and put that (upside-down) onto the sill. Who knows why?

Krik wrote about one time, when a brand new aid disappeared and she was determined to find it. Once out of the ear, if the battery isn't removed, these hearing aids emit a high whine, which continues 'til the battery flattens; this was often how we managed to locate it tucked away in drawers - or the linen cupboard – or wherever. This particular day Krik, after checking all the likely spots without success, suddenly had the bright idea it could have gone out with the rubbish.

Mum's food scraps were always wrapped in newspaper. An instinctive environmentalist, she never used a plastic bag – hated them. She always had a folded sheet of the Herald ready on the kitchen bench, where she would deposit anything destined for the bin. This included vegetable peelings etc. As soon as she had a small pile of scraps, she would bundle it up and immediately drop it into the wheelie bin near the kitchen door.

So there they were at the bin, Kriket diving in, lifting each bundle, holding it to her ear, carefully unwrapping it and sifting through the contents, then putting it aside to grab another one, with Mum at her elbow demanding to know why she was going through the rubbish. Even more annoying, she kept dropping the bundles back in with Kriket yelling at her to leave them alone. The deafness necessitated shouting:

'I'm looking for your hearing aid.'

'Why? It isn't lost?'

'Yes it is – that's what I've been looking for for the past half hour.'

'What? Have you? But - in the bin? Why?'

'Because I've looked everywhere else!'

'Well it won't be in there – that's ridiculous!'

And so it went, over and over, Krik desperately diving, Mum protesting, both jostling bundles of rubbish.

It didn't turn up and finally a letter came from the department, noting the multiple replacements and stating that from now on they would have to be paid for. The only solution would be for Kriket to remove it each night but this suggestion was met with complete refusal. Kriket explained that this was the fourth aid and the last free one - she hoped practicality would influence Mum, because she so disliked spending money on herself, but the only response was hot denial, accusations of being lied to and indignant protestations about being treated like an idiot.

As usual, in the face of such an onslaught, surrender was the only option and Krik had continuing, regular hassles.

~

Mum turned her television on at 6 p.m. each night. Nothing would induce her to watch during the day - this was being slothful and wasting time - although I regularly suggested it, because over time she stopped going into the garden as often and spent most of her time in her favourite chair on the verandah gazing out the window, often napping – always sitting upright.

To the last day she was in her house she refused with indignation the idea of taking an after-lunch nap. She had no notion that she often dozed off in her chair. I just thought she'd be more comfortable on her bed but apparently this was another sign of weakness - 'Days are for working.'

However, evenings were for relaxation so the T.V. went on between when she had her dinner at six p.m.and nine, when she went to bed.

Almost every night we'd have the same conversation.

'How do I turn the television on?' She'd wave the remote control.

'You press the red button...'

'Really? No-one's ever explained that before.'

She had no interest in changing the channel – insisted on the ABC - but it wasn't always very engaging for her so I would surreptitiously change it to lighter programs. She'd giggle at 'Two and a Half Men'. Without fail, when the boy sang during the intro, she would exclaim over his beautiful voice - how clever he was - saying she'd never heard him before. How wonderful for repetition to be ever-fresh! But sometimes she remembered how frequently she saw him:

'Goodness he's in a lot of programs, isn't he?

Then later on, preparing her for bed, the hearing aid tussle would begin. Various approaches were required.

'Could you take it out now so I can put it away before I go downstairs?'

'No, I'll do it in a minute. I'm right - off you go.'

'I'd like to put it on the side table so we can find it in the morning.'

'Well. I'll do that - I always put it in the same place. Off you go.' She'd be getting exasperated - time for a different tack.

'Also, you can't always remove the battery and then it might go flat.' I'd hope that a practical activity that she could recognise was a bit difficult for her would persuade. However, this could also lead to a whole dragged-out chat about the battery, which she mostly didn't remember being part of the procedure, so I didn't mention it too often.

If I could gauge it right, becoming 'Matron' occasionally worked. I'd try being brisk and matter-of-fact, gently taking hold of the tiny plastic handle with, 'O.K. Let's have the hearing aid' and she'd allow me to remove it with an acquiescent giggle. Other times the head would duck away and the hand would go up to cover the ear, which left me no choice. Persevering and therefore upsetting her, just when I wanted her to relax into bed, could open that other can of worms – the potential for a very restless night. It was that, or giving in.

My persistence, resistance or capitulation depended on the degree of tranquillity or agitation during the day, whether I was missing the beginning of a favourite T.V. show or just desperately wanting to have time alone with a good book!

I could always sneak up later and cruise around listening for the tell-tale whistle. However, there were times when she actually did remove the battery. It was all very unpredictable.

∼

Another initial pleasure was feeding the resident magpies, which she had begun many years earlier, taking great delight in setting mincemeat on the landing outside the kitchen door, where the birds had her trained to come every time they called.

Large quantities of mince would be bought each week but I took over some of the preparation, dividing it into portions before freezing, then defrosting a few lumps each morning because previously she kept the whole tray of mince frozen, so that each time she wanted to feed the birds she'd pop the lot into the oven to defrost in its plastic tray, often forgetting about it. When I first arrived it had taken hours to surreptitiously scrape the accumulation of congealed plastic off the oven floor and shelves.

The birds seemed happy to consume it in whatever form it was delivered – raw, half-cooked or frazzled with melted plastic. I allowed nature to take its course. Over the months Mum became erratic in the feeding until she seemed to forget about them and the clever birds adjusted, coming less often, until eventually they stopped nagging altogether.

~

Despite crazy talk and irrationality, it's important for us to always keep in mind that many dementia-sufferers don't lose their intelligence. Also, my Mum retained her sense of humour, which at times was a godsend and she was more than capable of having quite long conversations on many topics. She avidly listened to the radio news every morning and insisted on watching the evening news, although much of it went over her head. But if something caught her attention we could discuss it at some length.

Fortunately she had always been a very curious person, interested to see and hear new things. The fact that none of it was retained was completely irrelevant. Life had to be about being in the moment; good experiences are nurturing and who's to say what the unconscious retains?

~

Mum had two identical pairs of flat, navy shoes, an older pair that she had chosen herself, which had comfortably stretched to accommodate the shape of her bunions, finally developing a hole, and a newer pair that Richard and Soe had cleverly found and presented as a gift. They were in better condition.

Mum never realised there were four shoes and often could be found with two right (or left) shoes on, whichever she found first. One time, preparing for a physiotherapy appointment, running late as usual because of all the searches that were a part of every departure, she carried her shoes to put on in the car.

When we arrived and I prompted her to put them on we discovered she had brought two left shoes.

'I don't know,' I said with a mock sigh.

'Well! Neither do I!' Was the rejoinder. 'And if you find out – please don't tell me!'

We had lots of laughs.

Gradually, my list of care activities lengthened. The T.V. control was one. Some nights she managed to turn it off herself, others not; I would try to be there on time to check but sometimes I was delayed.

One evening I found her in a state because she couldn't turn her television off. I handed her the remote.

'You know, you can turn it off yourself – you just press the red button.'

'Oh no! Helen's told me I mustn't touch anything.'

'Well, I'm Helen and I promise you I have NEVER told you not to touch it. I encourage you to do it yourself.'

'Oh 'No!' Mum said, with a knowing grin. 'I don't mean THAT Helen.' She tapped me on the chest. 'I mean the OTHER Helen.'

'Well, I'm not sure about her.' By now we were both laughing. 'THIS Helen is going to say goodnight and go downstairs, O.K?'

'Right! Goodnight HELEN.' She followed me out into the kitchen, still laughing, holding the remote. 'Yes HELEN - Goodnight. Can I turn it off? Tell me, what do I have to do?'

'You press the red button. You can do it. You can do it every night, when you want to go to bed.'

'Oh - Goodnight, HELEN,' laughing and glancing over her shoulder as she pointed the remote.

There were times of insight - I remember her tapping the side of her head, looking at me pitifully, saying: 'I can't rely on this any more. You can't trust my brain.'

∼

One of my great supports throughout Mum's last years was

her wonderful G.P., Dr. Bill Wilson, a gem of the Old School. He still did house calls and Mum was on his regular three monthly roster, when he'd give her a check-up, renew the sleeping tablet prescription and give her a vitamin B12 shot. Her blood pressure never varied from 125 over 75.

Years before, when I lived so far away from her, he gave me his home phone number with the assurance that I could call at any time. Bless him! Although I'd never needed to call, such support makes a huge difference.

Despite her general physical strength and steadiness on her feet, I was always very aware of the potential for a fall, particularly as she tended to carry things up and down stairs not using the hand-rail. But - how can you anticipate it?

There we were one afternoon, both down in the garden, which was on a lower level than my abode, accessed by eight wide sandstone steps. Around 5 o'clock she announced she was going up for a cup of tea and started toward the steps, carrying her trowel and a bundle of weeds. Futilely I called out for her to please just hang onto the side and leave the weeds for me to bring up but off she went, scoffing as usual.

It was one of those slow motion moments. I began moving from further down so I was half-way across the lawn just as she reached the top, where I saw her stand up, straighten, then stagger. Legs flying, she turned a perfect backward somersault down the full flight of steps to land folded into the child's pose on the grass at the bottom, her forehead resting on the lowest step.

'This is it!' was my first horrified thought, as I bounded

up and crouched next to her. My mind was racing, trying to take it all in. As she rolled down I had seen the back of her neck catch on the edge of a step and I could see blood oozing. There she was, forehead on the back of her hands, face buried, quite still - but! - the next minute I heard:

'That's what I've been trying to AVOID doing!'

My thoughts tumbled. 'She's not dead!?!! But she must be so badly injured – I mustn't let her move! Keep her calm - settle her. DON'T PANIC!'

Suddenly she sat back onto her heels and began trying to stand. I insisted she stay there, lie sideways and wiggle all her extremities, which she did without any problem.

'Right! Now I'll have that cup of tea.'

Eventually I assisted her up the steps and into my room, where I phoned Dr. Bill, who recommended I keep her lying down, call an ambulance and definitely not give her anything to eat or drink.

More hassles with Mum. 'Don't be ridiculous! I just need a cup of tea!'

Very reluctantly she finally agreed, 'since the Doctor ordered it', so I made the 000 call.

Then. 'Oh no! I can't go to hospital!'

'Why?'

She was pulling at the elastic at her waist. 'I haven't got any of those ... you know ... little pants on.'

Her usual apparel was a comfortable pair of tracksuit pants with elastic waistband and sure enough, when I checked, she didn't have any knickers on but, I guess in compensation, I discovered she was wearing two tracksuit

pants, one on top of the other. She insisted I get her properly dressed before the ambulance arrived – Quick!

What could I do? Suppressing Dr. Bill's instructions not
to move her again, off came the two tracksuit pants, on
went a pair of my knickers and the cleanest of the trousers!

Feeling absolutely dreadful for refusing the now plaintive requests for a cup of tea, worrying that she would go
into shock, I can't overstate my relief when the ambulance
finally arrived.

I tried to help Mum deal with the confusion that began
to engulf her as the paramedics very efficiently strapped
her into a neck brace and immobilised her onto a stretcher.

Off we drove.

Always interested and apparently, unbelievably, feeling
no pain, she was most impressed that she was actually in an
ambulance! Pretty special!

I never want to have to repeat the evening that followed.
Her stretcher was placed in the queue of other stretchers
outside emergency and there we waited for the next two
hours until a bed finally became available.

Poor Mum! She kept begging me for a cup of tea and of
course she'd missed her dinner and was hungry as well.
She was so stoic – confused and terribly uncomfortable in
the neck-brace - but basically overawed by the strange environment, constantly asking me questions, wanting to know
who everyone was, what they were doing and where
she was.

Eventually she was moved to a bed where we waited
endlessly for a Doctor and when she was finally examined

X-rays were ordered, which meant I had to leave her, banished to the adjacent waiting room.

I discovered the treatment area could only be accessed by staff with an electronic key so I stationed myself next to the door and each time anyone entered or left I craned my neck to see if she had been returned.

At last I saw her. My request to go in was refused. It was a very simple matter to slip in behind the next staff member and if anyone noticed that I was back by her side, they didn't comment.

It was nearing midnight. She had no fractures or identifiable injuries apart from the graze on the back of her neck - was still talking to everyone - asking for tea! - and earnestly trying to understand the cognition questions put to her by the young, harried doctor.

Once again I explained she was deaf and had DEMENTIA and even I couldn't tell him what day it was by that stage, let alone the date! When he began suggesting that they keep her in overnight for observation I took a unilateral decision and told him very firmly that I would take full responsibility – that I was taking her home to her own bed. Her bewilderment was pitiful.

They insisted on taking her to the taxi in a wheel-chair, which amused her no end, then when she realised we were in a taxi cab she was highly impressed. An ambulance AND a taxi in the same night. The height of luxury!

At last – the cup of tea - the best she'd ever had I reckon. Eventually, after a bowl of soup, she began to wind down.

Her poor mind was turning cartwheels. I kept repeating how she'd done a backward somersault down the stairs in the garden, which necessitated the hospital visit but she absolutely refused to believe me.

As usual, my attempt to convince her to take a couple of painkillers was stymied. The half sleeping tablet, yes; any other tablet, an emphatic no! I knew her pain thresh-hold was very high and by then she was physically exhausted (she wasn't the only one!) so I tucked her in and crashed on a mattress outside her door.

I learned a few things through that experience:

1. My mother's bones were made of steel.

2. People with dementia are so relaxed they seldom suffer from shock.

3. I should avoid taking her to hospital again unless it was virtually terminal!

That turned out to be a prophetic thought.

While she didn't remember the accident and, miracu-lously, was left with minimal discomfort from bruising, the exotic experience seriously 'threw' her mind, resulting in several fraught days of agitation, bewilderment and general distress until we finally settled back into our routine and life resumed once more.

∾

In 2006, for those first few months after I had returned to live with Mum, another regular experience that used to set us up for hours of confusion and discomfort was going to the supermarket, an excursion which she insisted on being part of.

During the previous 18 months, she had managed quite

a lot of her own shopping but now I realised she had deteriorated markedly. I kept trying to convince her that I could shop for her, but it was useless.

All I could do was plan it for the morning, when she was usually somewhat more alert, which would also allow me time to get her back into a relatively calm head-space before nightfall.

She would slowly patrol the aisles, peering at everything, trying to read labels, picking up items she would never use, dragging the whole experience out into a major production, with me mentally measuring the serious impact the kaleidoscope of lights, colours, sounds and people was inevitably having on her mind.

Toilet paper was one of her foibles. I'd found more than a year's supply stashed in various cupboards when I first arrived but every week she'd insist on buying another six-pack. I'd surreptitiously remove unwanted items as fast as she was acquiring them until at last she'd let me take the trolley to the check-out, where she'd turn her attention to the other customers.

Loss of inhibition is another common symptom of dementia. A minor reason for not wanting to take her shopping was her propensity for making loud, inappropriate remarks such as 'Goodness that woman is fat!' or 'What IS she wearing?' and other derogatory comments.

I'd try to guide her into a queue near a mother and baby, if available - always a sure way for Mum to be totally absorbed. She loved children and babies, was great at communicating with them and they always responded to her.

Eventually – to my intense relief - after a few months, she relinquished the shopping trips.

For the demented, it seems that any change, e.g. going into strange surroundings, or even having visitors, can set off extreme reactions.

While Mum loved it when someone came to visit, the subconscious effort required to maintain conversation took great mental energy, often causing adverse reactions once they departed.

Our excursions were limited to short drives to local natural beauty spots – the beaches, Deep Creek, Narrabeen Lake and a long-time favourite picnic spot, Oxford Falls, which she had always said she wanted to be her final resting place. These were all old haunts and she loved re-visiting them, gently nurtured by Nature.

~

For most of 2006, I was able to occasionally go out in the evening, though I always returned before Mum's bedtime at nine.

As I left to go to a friend's exhibition opening late one afternoon, I made a mental note that when I returned I needed to put the garbage bin out ready for early morning collection. However, when I returned, to my surprise it was sitting on the kerb; Mum hadn't thought of this chore for months.

She greeted me, very excited and full of a story. Yes, she had gone to look out the gate just as it was getting dark and saw the neighbours' bins were at the kerb so she trundled ours out. Then some children had thrown a ball up onto her porch roof so she had climbed up to fetch it.

Also, a young woman had come to visit: 'She kept asking me if I was all right; I really don't know why. I can still climb a ladder without any problem. I have no idea who she was but she was very nice.'

Going cold at the thought I tried to elicit details, tactfully suggesting that climbing a ladder in the dark and walking on the roof probably wasn't such a good idea.

'Ah, I was very careful, I went down on my hands and knees,' she assured me.

Where was the ladder she'd used? Put away under the house of course. Puzzling!

Later, downstairs, I discovered a note from Chris, who lived across the road, asking me to phone her. She was quite shaken - had driven home with her kids just after dusk and when she slowed to turn into her driveway, her headlights caught what she thought was a white cat in the middle of the road.

She stopped, to discover my mother crawling across the road, very disoriented and gabbling about 'just going home'. Mum's pure white hair had been caught by the headlights! Chris, a nurse, gently and kindly led her back inside and settled her down.

Obviously, Mum had taken the bin out, then, becoming disoriented in the poor light, she very sensibly decided crawling was the best option to avoid tripping, so off she went, unfortunately, onto the road, away from the house rather than toward it. Amazingly, she'd dreamt up a dramatic story to tell me, weaving the random facts together.

That was the last time I left her in the evening. I also hid the stepladder behind the hot water system! I remembered it was only a few years before, when she was ninety, that she had come home from a neighbour's after babysitting to discover she had lost her back-door key. Ever-resourceful, she had collected the long wooden ladder from the side passage and climbed up through the open verandah window on the high side of the house. That ladder had been disposed of long since but I'd forgotten about the smaller one. I couldn't put anything past her.

~

During that first full year I would try to cue Mum about appointments, which I always scheduled for the morning. The following is a typical early scenario:

The night before I announced: 'Tomorrow morning you have an appointment to have your hair cut and permed. We'll leave here at about quarter past nine.'

Next morning, 8.15, as she was finishing her breakfast I went into her bedroom to find some decent clothes for her to wear. I lay them on her bed hoping she'd choose to put them on.

'I'm just taking Banjo for a walk. We'll be leaving at quarter past nine.'

'Right! I'll get ready then.'

Passing by on my way back at 8.45 I found her dozing on the verandah.

'We'll be leaving in half an hour'.

'Oh! I fell asleep!' She began climbing out of her chair.

'Never mind, there's still time,' I assured her as I shepherded her into the bedroom.

Returning at 9.05 I found her back asleep in her chair.

'Oh! Oh!' Time pressure meant she had to shuffle into the clothes, followed by much rummaging to find her powder – her lipstick – her shoes - the search for her bag, all the time with me grimly reassuring her that we still had plenty of time.

Then: 'We won't put your hearing aid in because you will be having your hair washed.'

I could see her beginning to worry. This wasn't a good start to a major excursion. Her hand went to her head.

'Oh, I should have washed my hair.'

'No, no, they'll do everything.'

'Are you sure? Well, I do have to take the hearing aid with me everywhere.'

The hearing aid went into the bag.

I made a quick call to the salon - we'll be there … soon!

Sitting on the bed, peering at the side table, she picked up her eye drops.

'Have you put them in this morning?' I asked. What possessed me? I still hadn't learned to avoid complicating such situations.

'Oh yes. I always do that straight after breakfast.'

(This was debatable but time was passing.)

'Well then, you don't need them now.'

'Yes! I need to take them with me.' The bag was beginning to bulge.

So, everything stashed, shoes on the correct feet, bottom teeth in, I dared hope we were finally on the way and urged her toward the door. But she baulked and headed for the bathroom:

'I'd better wet before I go.'

Into the bathroom - door closed. There followed a mumbling soliloquy interspersed with self-demands:

'Wet! Wet!' Then - much louder: 'I can't!'

'Never mind – just take your time.' (We were already late. What was another 5 minutes?) I heard the sound of running water – she'd turned on the tap to prompt her own waterworks. I headed into the kitchen for a glass of water.

Sip sip - 'WET!' she commanded. I quietly left her to it.

Finally! … Relief!

Throughout all this I endeavoured to remain casual and calm. (Grrrrr!)

At last we were both in the car, where she made a great show of trying to put on her seatbelt, which she allowed me to fasten in place - something she always remembered to prompt me to do. 'Don't forget to lock me in!'

'All set? Off we go!'

She suddenly sat back and emitted the deepest sigh. (Thought bubble - 'Oh! God! What now???') but, quietly,

'What's wrong?'

Another sigh, looked plaintively up at me: 'I'm turning into Grandma, aren't I?'

'Who? You? NEVER!'

Time for a quick hug and a laugh. Her natural sense of humour would always surprise me and this time, unknowingly, she completely defused the situation beautifully herself. It could have gone so very differently.

Before too long it became necessary to announce appointments allowing just exactly the right amount of time to get ready, find everything and leave, because increasingly, if I gave her too much notice, she spent the intervening time coming to me, asking if it was time yet, worrying that she was going to be late, restlessly putting clothes on and off.

I'd try to limit the searches by locating lipstick, teeth, hearing aid, etc. and putting them on her dressing table - which didn't always work because she could manage to relocate them all over the house in a very short time if the whim took her.

I really believe that once the information was received her sub-conscious innately understood not to let the thought go, knowing she would forget.

~

Something else I dealt with regularly were delusions, which, although a very common symptom of dementia that can be quite horrific for some, in Mum's case were often simply diverting.

Apart from the usual, such as ascribing perceived injustices to me, or accusations of telling lies, for some years she maintained a very persistent, regular hallucination; she'd see very well-dressed people, men, women and children walking up into the sky from under her house, floating over her garden and disappearing into the blue.

'There they are again! Can't you see them? They're dressed in their best; the women have hats on. Look there's a woman holding a child's hand. Up they go!'

She'd be entertained for an hour or more, watching them, describing their clothing. She'd insist they were coming out of my room so we'd both go down to look but on discovering they'd 'disappeared' she'd happily tell me they came out from 'somewhere else'. It was a mystery that was never solved but mercifully it didn't bother her.

One time I suggested that perhaps they were on their way to Heaven.

'Good Gracious, no! They're much too well-dressed for that!'

There followed a long discussion about suitable heaven-bent clothing, which she had definite opinions about. This sort of chat was straightforward - a 'talk- play' – light-hearted and fun, as any friends might have.

I asked if she thought they were ghosts but they didn't fit her idea of ghosts either. They looked too real, apparently.

Piles of clothes began appearing, draped across lounge chairs. 'This isn't mine. I don't know why it was in my room so I'll just leave it here for her to find.'

At first I suggested that this garment must actually be hers because, look, she had sewn it herself.

Pointless. The piles grew; I'd return a few to her drawers when she wasn't looking so there'd be something for her to find to wear but from then on furniture draped with clothes became the norm. She never seemed to fret about 'her' not collecting them, thank goodness! It fascinated me that Mum could create a new activity and continue to remember to repeat it.

~

Doors became a major problem. One of Mum's fetishes was closed doors. She HATED having her doors closed until bedtime. Even in winter I'd have a fight to shut them. She'd be huddled over her little heater, indignantly complaining about the cold but when I suggested the draught was from the open back door I was ordered to 'Leave it'.

During the early months she was capable of closing and locking all her doors after I left her each night, just before she went to bed. She usually just turned the keys, leaving them in the locks, which was useful from the point of view of not losing them but created difficulties for me.

I had a spare back door key but couldn't use it to access her place when there was already a key in the lock inside. A major problem arose when, although she was fine locking them at nine o'clock in the evening, she began to lose the ability to actually turn the key to unlock them in the morning.

Unlocking them had always been the very first thing she did as soon as she was out of bed every day. My practice was to go up through the back door to check her each morning just after seven until one morning, when I could hear her pottering in the kitchen with the door still locked.

We exchanged loud 'Good Mornings' through the door and when I pointed out that it was still locked I heard her fumbling at the key emitting little frustrated yelps.

'It won't work,' she yelled.

'I've got a key so if you pull yours out I can get in.'

More rattling: 'I can't - it's stuck!' She'd managed to jam it.

Great! Now what?

There ensued another long high decibel discussion with me yelling instructions and her protesting that it wasn't working, until – relief! - her key fell out. She was mainly amused that she didn't seem to know how to turn the key and I blamed the age of the lock causing stiffness so we laughed it off.

I appealed to her practicality and after several evenings of small skirmishes we reached a compromise; I would have the back door key and lock it as I left each night, leaving her in charge of the key to her front door. To avoid further problems I quietly removed the duplicate.

At times she'd go looking for this, wanting to revert to the old habits and I'd join her in the search before finally assuring her that I had my key so there wasn't really a problem. 'It'll turn up' usually settled things but I did get the evil eye on more than one occasion.

I HAVE mentioned how devious one becomes. As I slipped more and more easily into creating lies and fabricating scenarios I did sometimes worry about how adept I became. Was I becoming so practiced that it would form a habit and I'd behave this way with other people? However, I knew it was a necessary tactic for dealing with someone with dementia. (Fortunately, the habit didn't persist in later years.)

The front entrance to her house was a pair of old

wooden-framed double glass doors leading straight into her lounge-room from the street-level courtyard. These doors and their locks were to become an ongoing problem.

They both had sturdy barrel bolts top and bottom plus an old-fashioned internal lock with a large key. For a while she retained the capacity to lock her front door but the unlocking became impossible.

To save her realising this, I'd get upstairs earlier and unlock the front doors before she emerged. Eventually, the locking also was beyond her; she almost always pushed the barrel bolts into place but was usually content with giving the key a bit of a jiggle then walking away.

I'd go downstairs, wait until she was asleep and then quietly let myself in through the back door, turn the key and leave it in place confident that all was secure. This arrangement lasted several months.

Major dramas lay ahead.

~

As we moved through 2007, Mum's 98th year - my second full year with her - she began to slow down more and more, sitting for hours in the same chair, calmly gazing out from her glassed-in verandah that extended right across the back of the house. There was a lovely view down into the garden and out across the nearby beach to the sea with a park next door, so there was often plenty of activity to engage her. Because the house was built on a sloping block, the front was at street level but the back allowed for two storeys. My abode was under her back verandah.

At first I hadn't been allowed to do any gardening; she managed fairly well herself and I learned to be as adroit at making careful sorties in to tend various areas without her seeing, as I was at vacuuming when she had dozed off.

But her cognisance slowly dulled and she grew to accept me as the gardener. She would go out every day for a short period and busily pluck away at the increasingly unruly weeds, blissfully unaware of the minimal effect she was having, just happy to be among her plants. Her deteriorating eyesight - or was it lack of visual memory? - prevented her from seeing the neglect. (I wasn't the gardener she had been and I gradually converted her precious annuals beds into shrubs and ground covers, allowing certain areas to pretty much run wild.)

However, in her mind, she was out there constantly. Invariably, when my brother phoned she would blithely describe how she had spent the 'whole day' in the garden. I wrote to the girls:

'Yes, I feel sorry for Mum as well - she is truly just sitting, waiting, now - has been for around a year I reckon. She spends most of her time out on the verandah just staring out - and sleeping with head lolled - she is starting to forget about having cups of tea at ten a.m. and even lunch is being forgotten.

I don't think it'll be too long before I'll need to do most of these things for her. She even sometimes does let me make her a cup of tea and get her lunch! I've been helping quite a lot with the evening meal for a while now as well - I need to prompt her at every stage.

It's all perfectly natural - I just so hope that she can keep fading away gently – wouldn't that be wonderful? I sometimes feel guilty that I haven't spent enough time with her, just sitting, talking, though I do try to do that quite often. I still can't be sure what she really wants and am very mindful of not intruding (in her eyes.)

Although virtually every night she asks for help with the T.V., as well as organising her meal and seems happy to allow it, suddenly, one day, if I anticipate by starting to turn on her oven or get the vegetables out because I happen to be upstairs and it's about the right time, she will revert and accuse me of running her life, ordering me to 'Go home! Now! I don't need any assistance. What do you think you're doing?' and so it goes. I have to get out – and wait.'

∼

Mum always needed to use the toilet at least once during the night and to begin with it was a straightforward process where she would get herself up then return to bed and go back to sleep. However, even though it was adjacent to her bedroom, increasingly she began wandering the house after she'd used the bathroom.

I rented a commode to place next to her bed to save her having to walk anywhere but after I set it in place and showed her, she was totally insulted; demanded that I remove it to the spare room at once. I cancelled the rental.

There was no way I could describe the night wandering to her; I knew she'd deny it and accuse me of lying.

She became almost obsessed with knowing the time and never, ever lost the capacity to tell the time on the large wall clock in her lounge-room so, once up, there she'd go, turning on all the lights, which stimulated her brain and threw her mind into total confusion.

I'd hear her padding about and try to time my arrival so that she wasn't too far gone for me to lead her back to her room, where she mostly settled down again quite quickly. However, this gradually began to change and the nightly wanderings increased.

The whole experience of tending Mum as the dementia increased left me with a fascination for the amazing capacity of the brain. I sensed there was always that 'knowing'. I discovered that impossible tasks during the day became a piece of cake at two or three a.m!

One night I was suddenly woken in the wee small hours by loud male voices and heavy feet clomping around upstairs, light streaming from all the windows. I was used to her night rambling, when some lights came on but this was something new.

Stumbling up the stairs, hastily tying on a sarong I arrived in Mum's lounge-room to be confronted by my tiny, bewildered mother, barefoot, in her rather shabby, almost see-through nightdress with three large policemen walking around checking out all the rooms!

They had spotted her wandering along the main arterial road three blocks over and escorted her into their car. Though rather disoriented she was able to give them her name and address, thank goodness, so they delivered her home.

They told me the front doors were wide open. Of course she had insisted she lived quite alone, which was causing the police some consternation. Without her hearing aid she fortunately couldn't hear my side-of-the-mouth assurances that she did have a live-in carer so, eventually, after questioning me closely, they departed.

Time for a cup of tea over which I tried as best I could to unscramble her thoughts and parry her questions, I finally managed to get her back to bed.

Her story was that she suddenly found herself in a house down the street and it was so dark she couldn't find her way out.

Those 'nice men'. 'Really? Were they the POLICE?' had driven her home. 'Was that a POLICE car?' She had no idea why they had 'visited' and I didn't labour the point.

I guess the experience of three burly policemen and a ride in their car can serve to imprint a delusion. She appeared to have completely forgotten the police as she never mentioned them again and, as every dementia carer learns, you never remind someone with dementia about anything. It only causes distress and confusion. But the next day she insisted I drive her around the streets so she could show me this particular house she had been inside the night before, eventually identifying the one on the corner.

'Yes! There it is!' She declared that she needed to go and apologise to the owners. I invented an errand that prevented us knocking on the door at that time, saying we'd be able to do that later, assuming she'd forget, since by then her short-term memory had drastically reduced.

Hah! She clung to her story for several days, with me constantly heading her off, reasoning with her that these people we've never met would possibly be disturbed to hear that a completely strange woman had entered their home in the middle of the night.

'Best left well alone,' I told her, over and over, a point she could agree with, although she persistently worried at it.

I discovered that many of the tactics we use with toddlers apply equally well with the demented. During a chat with Richard one time after he and Soe had spent five days with her he told me they had found Mum's behaviour really difficult.

'You need to think of her as a three-year-old,' I told him.

'Hmmmmnnn. More like two!' was his rejoinder.

Diversion is a major tool, so I watched for the gathering restlessness, aware she was more than capable of going off on her own and when I thought she was working herself up again, I'd brightly suggest a short drive down to the lake, which always pleased her.

I took pains to avoid passing that house for several days until, very thankfully, that memory passed into the mists.

The police told me about the Wanderers List they kept at the station, so I organised Mum's photo and details to be put on file, determined that this was a precaution only - never going to be necessary. I just had to find a way to keep her in at night.

The front doors were the weak link. Easily fixed.

When the locksmith arrived next day to remove the old lock and install a Yale, I really had to fend Mum off. She took great offence, hassling and ordering him to leave, complaining that she knew nothing about needing a new lock.

I had explained the situation to him over the phone and warned him there might be trouble and he took the abuse in good part, finishing the job as quickly as he could.

At such times I resorted to the authority of my brother. If I told Mum that Richard had organised the locksmith, plumber, repairman etc., she usually grumblingly accepted it. A quick phone-call to Richard later put him in the picture so he could corroborate the story to Mum. He was always prepared to go along with whatever situation I invented - marvelous and essential support.

Obviously her unlocking abilities were unpredictable but I hoped a different lock and key would be more of a challenge. I still wanted to leave her 'in charge' of her front door key so, much against my will, I decided to exploit the fact that she had some awareness that she sometimes mislaid things. I would remove the key after sneaking in to lock the doors each night, then hide it behind the curtain on the adjacent windowsill, prepared to 'find' it with her the next morning if I didn't get there before her.

Knowing how obsessive she was about controlling her doors, I felt tremendously uncomfortable doing this but deceit had become second nature and her well-being was always the prime concern.

I also managed to introduce a couple of more respectable nightdresses. As with all her clothes, she was wearing everything out and refusing to replace garments, even when they became seriously bedraggled and had holes, so when necessary I bought new things and gave them to her as hand-me-downs, telling her they didn't fit me any more.

Time passed.

Then - an email to the family:

'Had a phone-call at five this morning - the police. Mum had gone walkabout again. Fortunately a man just down the road saw her (collecting his paper from his front garden) and she apparently told him her name so he called the police. I collected her in the car - gave her a cup of tea and she went back to sleep for a while. She was most upset with herself - knew what had happened - said she was going mad.

I had taken both the keys downstairs last night because she had been a bit twitchy so I wasn't taking any chances. I really thought I'd locked her in safely.

However, she had managed to undo the barrel bolts on both front doors and must have rocked them back and forth - just forced them open - broke the new lock.

I definitely need to make sure all her nighties are presentable! Fortunately she had a decent one on last night - it was inside-out - but!

It's been a while and it probably wont happen again in the near future but it's so unpredictable! Now she'll doze most of the day. She's definitely slowing down more but after her weightlifting training in the bath she is so strong!'

Back came the locksmith. He recommended a deadlock but I was reluctant to go that far, because I thought she'd be bothered by its different appearance, so another Yale was fitted.

I lit upon the idea of reinforcing the doors by barring them from the outside so when Mum wasn't looking I installed two sturdy screw-eyes and found a metal bar to slip through them.

So, there I'd be each night, lurking outside, avoiding the light spilling through the glass - she never drew her curtains - waiting until she completed her last little activities - checking things, wandering in and out, looking at the clock, - until finally the light would be turned off and I could slot the bar across. As with so much else I was dealing with, it came down to timing. I couldn't change her movements - I needed to adjust mine to each situation. I got better and better at disciplining myself.

~

The weight-training mentioned above came about as follows: The skin on one of Mum's shins was very thin, and she often knocked it, causing a nasty sore, which was difficult to heal. This time I was able to organise the wonderful White Nurses, who regularly came to dress it for her but being bandaged meant she couldn't shower, as was her custom. She needed to take daily baths with the leg elevated to avoid getting the dressing wet so I found a plastic stool to prop her leg on.

Mum took this all in and really understood. But when I turned up before seven next morning at her regular bathtime, my help was firmly rejected. She insisted that she could manage on her own and despite my trying several more times, she finally convinced me. I had to give up - having a hassle first thing was not a good idea at all.

Things progressed for several weeks. Eventually she was able to have a waterproof dressing so she could return to showering. I removed the plastic stool.

Then one morning I discovered the upholstered foot-stool from the lounge-room in the bath - soaking wet. Another family email:

'I jinxed the situation with Mum, saying she hadn't got angry lately. This morning I got ordered home again when I tried (once more) to point out that she didn't seem to be using both her eye-drops, because the level in one bottle is right down and the other is still almost full, although they were opened at the same time and she is supposed to put one drop from each in each eye.

'I do use them both. Don't talk to me - talk to the bottle. There's something wrong with it. I'm very careful about my eyes.'

'Yes, well that's why I'm mentioning it. I want your eyes to be kept as good as possible.' Blah blah - on it went.

So I backed off that and then (stupidly) I mentioned the saturated upholstered stool in the bath. While her leg was bandaged she couldn't shower (I tried to help her with this but she got up earlier and earlier) she somehow got herself into and out of the bath every day without help.

Try heaving yourself out of a bath with your leg up on a stool! She's effectively done a weight-lifting course over the past six weeks! However, for almost two weeks she has had a waterproof dressing and has been having showers so I removed the plastic stool. A couple of days ago, I found the upholstered one from the lounge-room out in the courtyard soaking wet; it had been raining so I imagined that she'd taken it out and left it in the rain – not totally unreasonable because she likes to rearrange things.

But no! It seems she has reverted to baths and using a stool! (I'd removed the plastic one. I also took the two leather stools that used to be in the kitchen and bathroom away ages ago because I'm trying to stop her climbing on them.) Honestly, it's exactly like having a toddler! Shame is you know a toddler is developing - just going through a stage. She's reverting - irreversibly.

Undeterred, she just used the upholstered one. I've now hidden it downstairs and put the plastic one back. I really don't want her to try to bathe this way - but - ?

Soooo (again stupidly - I was at a somewhat low ebb and that's always when I make mistakes!) I tried to remind her that she doesn't need to have a bath - she is having showers again now. Ha! What do I know? When am I going home - why do I lecture her?

Banjo and I went to the beach. Had made a hair appointment - fortunately for 11 - so there was time to let her forget all that before I got into the marathon …

'Which doctor are we seeing?'

'No, the hairdresser.'

'Ah! the doctor AND the hairdresser?'

'Noooo.' Then - the usual searches - powder, lipstick, comb, handbag ('someone takes all these things.') Then, the inevitable: 'I'd better wet'.

Tissues have to be loaded into the bag. Finally, we go!

Thank goodness she'd forgotten our tiff. I fully expected her to refuse to get in my car and try to catch a bus!

So - it's all go!'

~

The leg eventually healed relatively well, and the days and weeks passed, with me confident I had overcome the night escape problem - until the night she demolished the lot -

managed to break the new lock, bend the bar, prize out one of the screw-eyes and take off down the main road once more.

It was becoming embarrassing with the police (not to mention my loss of sleep with interrupted nights, trying to be alert to sounds of absconding.) There were plenty of times when she'd simply wander the house at all hours, requiring various degrees of persuasion back to bed. Who knew what whim prompted the need to walk out into the night?

Such night activity is called 'sundowning' and is quite common with dementia.

I'd previously resisted the locksmith's recommendation of a deadlock but I was now faced with the realisation that I had no choice but to create a solid security system and truly lock her in at night.

I wasn't prepared to risk her being able to find the key if I hid it; her brain seemed to become quite alert and be at its sharpest at the very time of the night when I was at my lowest ebb and the sleep interruptions were beginning to take their toll on me. I couldn't catch up sleep during the day as she did.

The idea of actually locking my mother inside her house appalled me. I felt I needed permission to take this step. Both Richard and Dr. Bill agreed with the decision and the locksmith returned.

While she was puzzled by the new lock, Mum accepted it, pleased that she could turn the handle to close it herself, thinking this actually locked it.

I took full control of the key. Basically, I just had to make sure that I was up really early each day to release the locks to avoid causing distress.

~

In May 2007, just before Mum's 98th birthday I wrote to my daughters:

'I've been having hassles with Mum today - being cold but refusing to put another jumper on. She goes and gets one of her lightweight sleeveless summer over-shirts — sometimes has four or five on - then still complains about the cold. I finally got something warm on her a short time ago. She's getting whackier and whackier!'

The above was common in winter. Every morning I'd find her in summer clothes and have great hassles convincing her into warm clothes, yet at two a.m., when that old brain lit up, all systems firing, and she decided it was breakfast time, she'd get up and dress properly in several layers of warm clothing. The lightweight night-dress - worn to bed all year round - was always underneath.

I became quite relaxed about her nightly security, although there were nights when, an hour or more after I thought she was sound asleep, she would waken and go out onto her verandah, which formed the ceiling of my room, and call out to me. She knew which window was directly above to call through to summon me with: 'Are you there?' and she quite often actually used my name then. I had no idea what triggered this - did she truly know who I was? I couldn't even try to find out.

I was relaxed, that is, until one night after a rather disruptive day leaving me feeling somewhat frazzled and very relieved to finally be in bed with my book. I was just in that lovely drifting stage between waking and sleeping, when suddenly an apparition appeared framed in the window at my feet!

'Hello!' Very jaunty.

I almost had a heart attack!

There she was, her old Sunday hat, complete with artificial rose, perched jauntily on her head. Was I dreaming? How was it possible?

Then the wild thought: *'She must have died and this is her ghost!'* After all we'd had discussions about suitable attire for Heaven and I truly believed it was completely impossible for her to escape. *'Oh God! I'm finally going crazy!'*

It transpired that she had given up on trying to open the doors so moved to the adjacent old sash window, which hadn't been opened for decades. The window was just a fixture - I believed it was completely immovable.

But she had managed to release the swivel catch, heave it up and climb over the window sill! She discovered it was raining so, to protect her hair, she climbed back in to retrieve her best hat off the top of her cupboard. Then in complete darkness, she made her way down the sloping side path off the courtyard, which had periodic very uneven sandstone steps, to come and visit me. All this she brightly told me as I shook myself awake.

That took a bit of sorting before either of us was settled once again. Next day I got her down into the garden, out of earshot, then with the aid of a hammer and a few four inch nails, I made sure the two potential escape windows adjacent to the doors were permanently closed.

All the other windows in the house opened over increasingly long drops due to the slope of the land and since she liked to have them open most of the time, I had to just trust that her common sense (*Oh! please?!*) would prevail and she'd remember this.

Finger-crossing time again!

~

In October, 2007, more than three years after first moving to care for Mum, I wrote:

'Mum had a fall in her lounge room the other afternoon, while I was out walking Banjo. She told me about it as soon as I got back. Has wrenched the top of her right leg and has pain when she walks but seems to be able to sit down without any discomfort.

I've rented a walker for her but (of course!) I'm having great trouble getting her to use it - also, trying to get her to rest the leg and not go up and down stairs etc. Problem is she is liable to have another fall. We discuss this and yes! she agrees and then blithely trots off (or rather, limps off).

Dr. Bill came a few days later and when I told him he suggested an x-ray, just to be sure - said people can walk around with a broken hip! (Ye gods! I felt awful, assuming from her movements etc., that it was just a soft tissue injury!) So we organised that for the afternoon.

After the usual protracted departure we were standing in the foyer of the building, waiting for the lift to go up and have the x-

ray, Mum actually using her walker (her 'horse' as she calls it)
and she suddenly said:

'Make it stop!'

'What?'

Holding her head in both hands: 'It's all going round
and round.'

Poor sweet… I hate to see her distressed like that.

I dropped the x-rays up to Bill's office and he contacted me
later on to say all was well. Thank the gods! Of course, she was
totally bamboozled by the experience and we had a messy evening.

'Why are you trying to confuse me? - I KNOW they are
coming home - what am I going to feed them?' etc. etc.'

Many nights we had that conversation – she'd be
preparing dinner and fretting about how many to cater for.

One night it was a different question, which threw me.

'When is Laurie coming home?

She hadn't brought up my long-dead father before. How
to respond? Tell her the truth and risk causing grief and
distress? Tell a fib and say he wouldn't be coming tonight?
But my father never went anywhere, was always at every
meal and this was something she might well remember, so I
risked being caught in a real lie, as opposed to the
numerous innocent times when she accused me of fibbing.

I decided this was a time for honesty so put my arm
over her shoulder to try to soften the blow. I gently said:

'You see Edna, Laurie is with your mother.'

Quick as a flash: 'What?… My mother's dead! You mean
… HE'S dead?'

'Well, yes, he died many years ago.'

I braced myself to offer comfort - to plunge into a maelstrom of explanations …

'Really? And I haven't even missed him!'

Relief! We joked that she definitely didn't need to do extra vegetables for Laurie.

~

A vital key to staying on some sort of even keel and coping with the relentless repetitions (not to mention the dramas) was keeping in touch with other people. I did have a few lovely Sydney friends as well as a couple of cousins, who I tried to see occasionally, plus I kept in touch with many distant friends.

Of course my movements were somewhat limited but I was terribly lucky that my mother never deteriorated to the point where I had to be vigilant absolutely all day. I joined a small private gym, where I spent two hours a week, as well as a book club, which provided another short regular outing.

I felt fairly comfortable leaving her for up to three hours at a stretch between mid-morning and early afternoon. This meant I could even sometimes get down to the local cinema for a matinee. I spaced outings so that I wasn't gone on consecutive days and Mum was by nature a very undemanding person - except at the times when she became agitated and shrill over some imagined situation she reckoned I was responsible for.

Essentially, by keeping my distance for a part of each

day, even when I was around the house, she remained fairly self-sufficient emotionally.

Neither of us had ever suffered from loneliness and she was never a very demonstrative mother. Ours hadn't been a particularly hugging family, although I gave her a hug and a kiss on the forehead before she went to bed each night.

Various friends from Queensland periodically came for short visits, which was delightful for me. They would sleep down in my abode while I used Mum's spare room every night, although I took care to go there and leave while she was asleep to avoid explanations and confusion.

She always enjoyed socialising with my friends, who took her ramblings in good part. I remember she decided one was her cousin, calling her 'Cousin' throughout the visit. Another friend, Roz, told me how Mum had sidled up to her and quietly asked if she knew 'that woman living downstairs' and 'how long would she be staying?'

I had also joined a Dementia Carer Support Group, which was a true godsend. The fortnightly meetings allowed a dozen or more carers to 'vent', cry and get advice and input from the only people who really understand what living with a dementia-sufferer entails. At my first meeting I remember the hilarity in response to my anxious query if anyone else had found it necessary to lie and become devious.

One carer friend in particular, Lynn, a veteran, who cared for her husband with multi-infarct dementia for almost 12 years, became a valued confidant.

At around five on many afternoons we'd be on the phone, having another 'creative whinge', as Lynn called it.

It was a chance to provide an ear for each other. Not advice, just understanding. Such support is seriously essential for a carer. Alzheimer's is called the 'long goodbye' and the toll it takes on carers and families can be devastating.

Over the years that I was involved I came to know quite a number of carers, both during and after their commitments and I noted the very high proportion of them who soldiered valiantly and lovingly for years and years, only to be diagnosed with cancer once they were a 'graduate' as we called them - once their dependent had died and the responsibilities were lifted.

It's incredible how resilient people can be while they are entrenched in the daily demanding grind, when they are so needed, constantly under severe stress, only to succumb physically once they have been released. So cruel. I'd put the proportion at well over 70%.

I was always grateful that Mum merely had senile dementia, which could be thought of as a relatively natural part of the ageing process. My problems and experiences were extremely small compared to those of so many I met and came to admire.

My son, Matthew, was also able to come for visits from northern N.S.W. Kriket and Mark had moved to the U.K. so all communication with them was via email. But Richard and Soe came at Easter and Christmas each year to stay for about five days, which enabled me to take time off to travel to visit my older daughter's family in Central Queensland.

Richard's condition, inclusion-body myositis, a rare inflammatory disease causing incremental muscle wasting, naturally limited their visits, as it was extremely uncomfortable for him to be away from his own purpose-built environment. I was so very grateful for these breaks.

While I didn't find caring for Mum particularly onerous and I felt I managed the unpredictable situations and frustrations reasonably well, I always remained aware of the possibility of becoming overstretched. I tried to pace myself and knowing I had a short break on the horizon really sustained me.

~

My mainstay sanity tools were the radio (blessed ABC) the phone, my computer (both essential for keeping in touch with distant friends and family) music and books, plus walks on the beach and being with dogs.

I almost always managed a quick swim every morning after breakfast, a precious half-hour stolen when Mum was usually happily ensconced in her chair, finishing her pot of tea. This brought me in contact with a number of 'regulars', many walking their dogs, so Banjo and I could both socialise.

I did quite a lot of knitting and some sewing. I'd naively imagined before I moved down that I'd finally get a chance to get into some of my own larger creative projects, which I'd delayed for years because of the demands of work but this was actually a ridiculous notion. I couldn't start anything requiring quiet, or concentration, or prolonged application. Mum would inevitably find me and take great interest, asking endless questions, or I'd be required to help her answer the phone or unravel some other domestic situation. I didn't need any extra frustration!

One of the two major joys that Mum had over those last few years was music, when I'd play old tapes and vinyls - music from her youth. I discovered music is an incredibly valuable tool when working with people with dementia.

Dr. Oliver Sacks suggested, '*It really is a very odd business that all of us, to varying degrees, have music in our heads*' and this definitely applied to Mum. We'd sing all the old songs from her early years, all the words deeply embedded, never to be forgotten.

I remember coming across her perched on a wall in the garden one day and decided to undertake an experiment. There was a poem I'd heard my parents quote all my life. I began: 'I wish I was a rock…' and immediately she picked it up, speaking in the slow drawling voice with the burred accent of my Great-grandfather Podmore, a Yorkshire gardener, who had taught it to her as a child. He emigrated with his family when my maternal grandmother was three.

> '*I wish I wur a rock*
> *A-settin' on a hill,*
> *A-doin' nuttin' aaaaall day long*
> *'cept just a-settin' still.*
> *I wouldn' eat,*
> *I wouldn' sleep,*
> *I wouldn' eeeeven wash!*
> *I'd jes' set there a miiiiillion years;*
> *An' rest meself, by gosh!*'

'Goodness! Where did that come from?' She laughed. 'But that's exactly how I feel!'

From then on, as with a toddler, I'd often prompt her to recite this, bringing her pleasure, eliciting the same triumphant reactions you'd expect from a small child. Sometimes the simplest things bring the greatest reward.

The other constant joy was Banjo, my little Jack Russell cross, plus two other dogs that I regularly minded for a friend.

The 'two Bs' (Barney and Benjy) were often my mental saviours as well, because I'd adopted Banjo as a seven-year-old dog and he'd had a pretty awful early life, which left him with some quite serious mental issues of his own - real depression. The two Bs were normal - demonstrative enthusiasts of life - always ready for action.

Banjo would perk up when they were around, even sometimes playing with Benjy but he mostly preferred to be by himself, curled up in a corner, except at the end of each day, when he'd choose to sit with me just before I fed him. Since routine ruled the rest of the household, every day had much the same rhythm; this suited him beautifully.

However, he was truly sensitive to people's moods and often quietly sat near Mum on the verandah, where she'd chat away to him as he blissfully dozed.

December, 2007 brought daily thunderstorms, which terrified poor Banjo.

I wrote:

'Banjo has gone (more!) whacky lately, as well as Mum. (She was up and showered and dressed, with all lights on, radio blaring and jug boiling at one this morning.)

*He won't get onto the couch or chairs or beds any more - abso-
lutely refuses. He's taken to climbing up to sleep on shelves e.g.
the bottom shelf in the bathroom on top of the towels (very
narrow, so legs hang out) my computer keyboard, the table next to
the computer which is overloaded with my little piano keyboard
and radio as well as various piles of papers (most end up on the
floor.) AND - his favourite place, where he takes himself off to
sleep every night at present - on top of the junk on the bottom
shelf of the old tray-mobile in the laundry!*

*Plus, he doesn't come to tell me about his dinner in the
evening any more (the only time he used to seek me out and actually want to talk, as you know.) So we live at arm's length
(except, of course, when there's thunder - THEN he's sitting on
my lap.) Come to think of it, maybe he only has one slice of
'friendly-cuddle pie' per day and now that he uses it up in the
storm he hasn't got any left for dinner time. That might
explain it!*

*I don't know whether the daily thunderstorms have done his
head in as well! IS THIS HOW HE WILL BE FOR THE REST
OF HIS LIFE??? What have I done to him? Between him and
Mum they're doing MY head in, that's for sure! I worry! Thank
the gods the two Bs are here today! They are so NORMAL!! Here
they are sitting at my feet as I write.'*

Footnote: Banjo lived for about four years after Mum
died and he steadily developed all her symptoms, dementia
eventually completely ruling my life once more. I used to
joke that I truly suspected her spirit had taken him over - a
bit of 'Mother's revenge'? In any case, the experience with
Mum sure served me well as an apprenticeship for dealing
with his affliction.

~

An avid Radio National listener, one day I heard a discussion about brain donation. It seemed that brain donations must be organised through a separate register from other organs and any brain, no matter how old, is welcome.

Mum had always very firmly stated that she would be happy for someone to have any part of her once she died, if it was of use; we had had many such discussions over the years, so I decided to contact Dr. Bill and ask his opinion. He agreed that she had told him the same thing. Also, that, despite her dementia, if I chatted to her and she understood and agreed, it would be ethical to register her.

One day when we were down by the lake one of her regular topics arose. What was going to happen when she died? Death was never a taboo subject in our family. I assured her that Oxford Falls was still there and we chatted about how she and Richard had taken Laurie's ashes up there.

Many years before my father had also buried their two dogs in the bush there (probably illegally?) but this was a comfort to her. It got a bit sticky when I realised that she expected to be buried as well. I explained that going into a public area with a coffin and a front end loader was pretty much out of the question - the Council might have something to say about it. The best we could do was scatter her ashes.

There was a pause '…You mean I'd be burnt? … No! I don't think I want to be burnt!'

'Yes, well, cremation - just as Laurie was. That's the only

legal way you can choose your last resting place. Otherwise there's the cemetery.'

Hmmmnn … Lots of round-and-round discussion re the pros and cons of body disposal choices and finally, after a bit of giggling she decided this would be O.K. specially if the alternative was to be buried in a 'graveyard'. She didn't fancy that notion at all.

She seemed really quite lucid so I broached the idea of brain donation, reminding her that she had always wanted to pass anything useful on. I pointed out that because of her advanced and amazing age, there probably wouldn't be much call on any of her organs but she was in the minority of people living into their late nineties and medical science would value the contribution of her brain.

This appealed to her practical side and she quite happily agreed for me to obtain the forms and organise it. She was quite tranquil and unusually engaged. Her final satisfied comment was:

'That must be why.'

'Why what?

'Well, you tell me I'm 98. I must have got so old in order for doctors to be able to examine my brain!'

As my friend Lynn used to say - sometimes the Christmas lights came on!

The family all agreed so I followed through and filled out the forms.

~

There was no point in hankering for any changes in my

situation but I daydreamed about going over to Wales, where Kriket and Mark had moved to two years before.

An email to them in late 2007:

'Well, there's no trip planned in any way of course, but back in April I laid a foundation for the dream - decided to apply for a passport. Wishful thinking in some ways but they do last for ten years!

I'm still trying to find a way for someone to live in for a period - not so easy, of course - and there'd be stuff to sort before we could do it, like getting the upstairs carpets cleaned and the place a bit spruced up, not to mention gauging Mum's demeanour.

She still does her 'secret Nan's business' in the bedroom - although she doesn't have the bucket any more. I'm really not sure how she manages but there are sometimes newspaper-wrapped bundles behind the door plus drips and blobs across the carpet where she walks. She doesn't always take the bundle to the bin (yes, any bin still does!) and leaves it on the floor in the bedroom.

I minded the two Bs all last week for John and this presented problems. I found shredded newspaper spread all over the floor one day (can only imagine the fate of the contents! Yuk!!!). Benjy took to racing upstairs and checking it out first thing every morning, so I had to get in there fast before him each day after that!

I'm working up to broaching the commode suggestion again. I must say it's quite remarkable that she isn't the least bit incontinent yet. Everything is controlled. It's just the choice of deposit sites that's the problem! That can't be too hard to sort out! Can it?

So - I'm working on everything - thinking that it will be two years at Christmas and she's charging on physically. I'll need to take more than just a few days off here and there; need to organise some sort of respite help other than Richard and Soe because that's not entirely guaranteed into the future. It must be increasingly difficult for Richard to stay here I imagine. We'll see. I've definitely put it out there!'

'Secret Nan's Business' ... Kriket had coined the phrase. Unfortunately whenever Mum needed to 'pass a motion', as she called it, rather than the toilet, she chose to use a bucket lined with newspaper. This was permanently stashed behind her dressing room door.

Of course, she believed that no-one would know. The problem was that she wasn't always completely successful when wrapping her bundle up (the bucket washing was pretty arbitrary as well) so when she carried the package outside, she often managed to drop bits, invariably treading in them, necessitating much carpet spot-cleaning.I could never cajole her to use a plastic bag – she absolutely hated plastic - always the environmentalist. I guess she knew she shouldn't put newspaper into the toilet (thank heaven for small mercies!) Hence the trip to either the kitchen bin or the main wheelie bin outside.

Preoccupation with bodily functions can be one of the more debilitating symptoms of dementia. She was obsessed about becoming constipated - utterly determined to avoid it.

The overwhelming need to keep control of all aspects of her life was never extinguished. She would sometimes confide in me her horror of ever wetting the bed. I acquired some adult disposable continence pants as a precaution, dreading the thought that I'd ever have to ask her to use one. (I never did.)

At best, it's a terribly delicate subject to broach and I squibbed for a long time but eventually I did question her (after having to scrub the carpet several days running) to be told very crossly that she couldn't use the toilet because she needed to SQUAT and a bucket was more convenient because it was low to the floor.

'It won't come out when I sit on the toilet.'

I tried placing a low stool in front of the toilet at the same height and demonstrated how you could squat with your feet on the stool and knees up high but this was dismissed out of hand. Her system worked perfectly well and she saw no reason to change it.

'I need a hole - dig me a hole, then!' was her retort!

Eventually I did manage to wean her off the practice to the degree that the revolting bucket was removed. But, behind the door of the dressing room had to be the spot so I put a large sheet of polythene plastic down for her to spread her sheets of newspaper on. I also propped a sign against the wall behind the door asking her to 'please try to use the toilet' written in large letters. I don't know why I bothered but I really wanted to be able to hire a relief carer at some stage.

Who can still squat at 98? My mother could.

∼

Christmas was coming and I wrote: 'Have been pricking my conscience a little, thinking I should tart up Mum's place because *she used to love having Christmas decorations. Not sure if I'll succumb though - feeling too tired.*

However, I might have told you I bought a ticket for her to go to the Messiah, not sure if she'd be up to it on the day, of course but I took the chance. I knew I couldn't do it alone so I invited Robbie and we went on Sunday.'

The previous year I had the great joy of participating in the annual combined choirs performance of the Messiah in the Sydney Town Hall. Not long after that I had to forgo all evening activities, so I couldn't be in the choir any more but hoped to attend a performance the following year.

The problem was it would be in the afternoon and I'd be away too long to leave her. I knew Mum would love the experience too, so I recklessly decided to attempt to take her to the matinee.

This was going to be the most ambitious excursion I had attempted so it was planned like a military exercise. By then I was fairly practised at organising departures, timed to prevent her obsessing about going, gauging just enough time to dress and prepare her to leave (allowing for finding all the mislaid necessities.) My cousin Robbie agreed to be assistant.

Living locally Robbie was a regular visitor and one of the four people Mum always knew, so I was confident she would make the outing even more enjoyable for Mum. (The other people never forgotten were Richard, Soe and my son, Matt, all of whom she genuinely recognised even months after last seeing them.)

Despite my misgivings I was really looking forward to it.

I planned to tell her at around 11.45 a.m. with the departure time scheduled for 1 p.m. I needed to get her through an early lunch without rushing. Earlier I had ironed a couple of 'best' dresses, hardly ever worn these days, to give her a bit of choice and then looked for her slightly decent pair of flat navy shoes to clean them. I found the right shoe - no sign of the left.

She was out on the verandah snoozing (bolt upright as usual) and sure enough there was the left shoe on her right foot with the old left shoe on her other foot.

She woke up when I tried to prize it off so, even though it was a bit earlier than planned, I decided to divert her, saying:

'We're going to hear the Messiah in the Town Hall in the city.'

'The Town Hall? Good heavens! I don't mix in THOSE circles!'

'No, It's like a concert - lots of different people will be there.'

'But I haven't got a hat!'

'You don't need a hat - it's not church.' Then, 'I need the shoe you've got on your right foot so I can clean it.'

'Oh? What about the other one?' taking the old left shoe off.

'I've already got the other one.' (sometimes I'm soooo stupid!)

Puzzled look; 'But it's here' (pointing at her left foot.)

'Ah! No - that's from your other pair. See this is a left shoe too and I've already got the right one here.'

Inwardly kicking myself, I showed her the shoe in my

hand, thinking, *'I must be mad! Why do I start these things? Why didn't I just take both of them?'*

I think I was a little anxious about the wisdom of this excursion and was obviously too focussed on the outing to anticipate a drama and head her off.

'I haven't got another pair.'

'Yes you have – see? I've got two shoes the same and you've got one of the other ones.'

'That's three shoes, not four.' Logic had jumped into this bizarre exchange; no alternative but to produce the old right shoe. Hah! stupid! It could be ANYWHERE! I'm rummaging around, losing time, she's following me saying she doesn't have two pairs; why would I tell her such a thing, why do I try to confuse her? Do I think she's stupid?

Seeing all chance of any outing rapidly dissipating I abandoned the fourth shoe search and moved to my 'retreat' tactic.

'I'm just going to get these cleaned so they'll be ready for you'.

'Why? Where am I going?'

And so it went. Beginning to truly regret the whole plan, I took off downstairs.

So did she, one shoe on and one bare foot, dot and carry.

'I don't have two pairs of shoes … '

'O.K. Just come back upstairs. I'll get your lunch so you can be eating it while I do this.'

It worked. Finally we were getting it together. She was pretty much being stuffed into her clothes by me when Robbie arrived. 'Where's my lipstick?' - search around -

can't find hers - can't find my old one that I brought upstairs last time hers went missing.

Robbie and I insisted that we weren't wearing any so she didn't need to, which she very reluctantly accepted. Then: 'These shoes aren't right. I need to wear high heels with this dress'

I'd removed all her high heeled shoes after we had a terrible run-in one morning when I caught her in one high heel, one flat, bobbing up and down around the house, with me desperately following her, trying to get her to just sit down. I did lose it that morning: when she accused me of treating her like a three-year-old I told her to stop behaving like one. (THAT had been an interesting day!) We managed to convince her that flat shoes were definitely the best option - again - that was what Rob and I were wearing.

'What about stockings?' None of us had worn stockings for years. Where was she dredging all this from?

'No! no! No stockings.' I was totally forgetting all the strategies. The Golden Rule - NEVER CONTRADICT - had gone out the window.

'But I can't go out without stockings … you HAVE TO wear stockings to those places'

Keep calm, Helen, I reminded myself. *You really thought this was a good idea? Are you mad?* Rob and I rolled our eyes at each other.

After making sure the hearing aid was in place, FINALLY we were on our way.

I dropped my passengers off outside the Town Hall and Rob took her inside to find our seats while I parked in the underground car-park across the road. I had arranged to meet two other friends and they were already seated with her when I got inside, making a lovely fuss of Mum, adding to her excitement, so impressed that she was 'in the Town Hall!'

I could hear her customary loud comments as she looked around and I soon realised she was so overwhelmed by it all that I no longer existed in her consciousness. All I got was a vague, polite smile as I sat down next to her before she turned back to Rob.

The loud remarks about 'really being inside the Town Hall - in the city!' and 'Heavens! So many people! Why are they all here?' were drawing sidelong looks from adjacent seats.

I'd warned Robbie that I couldn't predict how she'd cope; we most probably would have to leave before the end but my fingers were tightly crossed that she'd settle down - *Soon! Please!* - and we'd at least hear part of the beginning of the performance.

Then, the choir in place, the orchestra on the stage, in walked the first violin. The audience began clapping.

'Who's that?' (very loudly.)

'The lead violin.' (just loud enough, hoping I only needed to say it once.)

The orchestra began tuning.

Head cocked - 'What's that noise? Has it started?'

'They're tuning their instruments.' (I could sense the people behind us raising their eyebrows and sighing.)

'Well!' - even louder and very huffy - 'Wouldn't you have thought they'd do THAT before they go on stage?' (By now, the hostility from the adjacent seats was palpable and

I was calculating how soon I'd have to remove her.) My apologetic smiles weren't allaying the restlessness.

Finally the conductor arrived and Mum enthusiastically joined in the clapping. Then Handel began to work his magic. I could hardly believe it! She sat, completely entranced, throughout the entire first half.

Interval came and she was totally happy. She had latched onto Robbie as 'her person' - didn't only remember she was her niece - kept introducing her to everyone nearby calling her god-daughter (which Robbie was but Mum had previously ALWAYS remembered Rob's name; I thought the god- daughter fact had long been forgotten.) I had become this stranger sitting next to her and she kept asking Rob to introduce us! During the second half she began asking who she had to give her money to:

'I haven't paid: who do I pay?'

(Oh! Lordy! Keep calm - remember - you're here to enjoy yourself.) Rob and I kept exchanging glances.

During the Alleluia chorus, when everyone stands - gooseflesh stuff - I placed my hand on her back, encouraging her to rise with us. Of course she recognised this and she was truly rapt; actually grabbed my other hand and held on!

It was raining as we left so we decided it would be quicker to walk her straight to the car. All the way across the road, with Rob and me on either side of her, she kept thanking me profusely (still the kind stranger from the seat next to her.)

I was so exhilarated that we'd been able to stay for the full performance, I must have been feeling sentimental, delighted about the success of the afternoon. Without think-ing, I explained I was actually her daughter.

'Oh!' She giggled. 'I thought you were just a nice kind lady helping an old woman!'

Suddenly she stopped and stared sideways at me, clearly suspicious, 'You're my daughter?'

Whoops! I'd dropped myself into a potentially fraught, protracted interchange but fortunately the conversation disappeared immediately because the pedestrian lights changed. I was saved from having to answer, as we hustled her onto the far footpath.

By then, her poor mind was reeling from maximum overload. After the wonderful atmosphere in the audito-rium, the crowds of hurrying people against a backdrop of surging traffic completely overwhelmed her. She hadn't experienced any form of crowded place for over a year.

But her natural curiosity bubbled out as we moved into the lift and began going down. She loved it, as excited as a child, totally bamboozled by this multi-layered building full of vehicles. 'All underground? Goodness!'

I'd disappeared again. She showed great surprise when I put her in the passenger seat and got behind the wheel. I was thanked several times. 'How did you find this car? Did you just choose one?' Then, craning back, in a stage whisper to Rob,'Why are we going with HER?'

The movement of the car, negotiating the spiral ramp, up and up, to finally emerge into the city streets, surrounded by tall buildings and full-on traffic, completely undid her. The mind had lost all reference points: 'Are we still underground? I can see lots of tall trees. Where are we? Where are we going?'

The loss of touch with reality required a constant running commentary all the way home. Despite my delight that she had been so enthralled and we had actually stayed the course, I was once again beginning to question my decision to take her, foreseeing days of endless hassles and total disorientation. I doubted whether the experience could compensate.

Of course, when we got to the door:

'Why are we here?'

'You're home.'

Turning back toward the gate, she protested in a very quavery voice, 'No ... I used to live here ... but I don't any more.'

The rain wasn't helping.

At last I managed to coax her inside with the promise of a cup of tea 'before we move on home'.

It had been a long day - fraught at times - but excellent! The evening was something of a haze but before she went to bed, she finally seemed to register where she was (thank the gods!) and, best of all - a small miracle - when I turned up next morning, she greeted me with a brilliant smile:

'That music! Wasn't that a wonderful concert!?'

Joy! We were actually able to talk about it for a few minutes. The power of music! Needless-to-say we never could discuss it again but retaining it overnight was amazing.

～

Richard and Soe spent Christmas 2007 with Mum, giving me a whole week's much-needed respite. They noticed a greater deterioration in her.

They were always wonderfully supportive of me, phoning Mum regularly, though this now had to happen through me, because she increasingly found it difficult to use the receiver on the regular phone. I'd have to hold it up to her ear. This became more complicated because she then developed the habit of removing her hearing aid as soon as I presented the phone. So we installed a conference phone, which Mum never understood how to answer or disconnect but which she could successfully hear and talk on.

Richard and I would arrange a time that suited me to be available. Before every call I needed to re-explain that there was no receiver and all she had to do was sit in the chair and talk normally, then each time a call was finished we'd have the conversation about this amazing modern invention and she'd insist on me showing her which buttons did what so that she could manage alone next time.

Her deterioration meant I didn't have to be quite so sneaky, but I was very aware that, while she no longer seemed to notice when I did housework - I could now openly do chores in front of her - there would be reminders of how she had been in the past. Out of the blue, I'd get a comment such as, 'You keep making things neat! You think that's important?' Subconsciously it definitely still irked her.

Another time, she walked past me when I was vacuuming, apparently without even noticing. A little later, when I joined her on the verandah, she asked me whether the woman doing the cleaning had been paid!

In February, 2008, as I entered my third year with Mum I wrote:

'Mum had to have her last two teeth (the lower front ones) out on Tuesday. I noticed her wincing when she was eating. She didn't tell me of course but I discovered they were both really wobbly and giving her pain.

The dentist promised to add new ones to her plate on the same day and it worked out well - that is, once we got there! Had to be there by 10.30 so I organised her and set her up with a cup of tea at quarter to 10.

Then I discovered she didn't have the bottom teeth in but after a bit of a search, thank goodness!, I found them stashed in the linen cupboard. I put them in the bathroom, telling her they were ready for her to pop in after cleaning her teeth. When I returned fifteen minutes later to take her, she was still sitting on the veran-dah, sans teeth - had totally forgotten we were going out, of course.

Into the bathroom – no teeth.

'Where's your bottom plate?'

'I haven't seen it'.

'But I gave it to you 15 minutes ago. Where have you put it?' My tone was rising – control, Helen, control.

'No , you're wrong! I didn't put it anywhere; I haven't seen it at all.' Her tone was echoing mine.

(Give me strength! Not now - please!) Stupidly, more shrilly - we're going to the dentist - sans teeth is NOT an option. 'Yes, you have - it MUST be here!'

That did it.

The hand thumped down on the sink. She turned and eyeballed me: 'Look! I didn't have it at breakfast.'

'I know you didn't!' (somehow she could remember breakfast but not 15 minutes ago!) 'I just GAVE it to you.'

I'm such a slow learner! That was it. Small as she is, she's strong and, as you know, when she becomes feisty she's formidable! She grabbed my arm, bundled me out the door and slammed it in my face.

So, off I went, searching, searching. Time was passing; quick call to the surgery. Sorry, running late. No problems, he was too, thank goodness. Back to looking, looking.

I thought she might have shoved it into the drawer in the bathroom (seem logical?) so, when she finally came out, in I went - but - no teeth anywhere… (don't panic!…? Of course, panic!) If we'd been going anywhere else it wouldn't have mattered but the bottom plate was the one requiring adjustment after the extraction.

I finally calmed down, joining her in the bedroom, desperately trying to think of the key question to trigger her memory without raising the ire. Looked at her. The plate was in her mouth!! I didn't ask!

But I got her out to the car quick-smart.

We got to the dentist just on 11 and all went well. Had to hide a laugh when he asked her if she had been having pain with the two teeth, which were really very wobbly:

'How do you mean - pain?'

'Well, did you need to take aspirin?'

It was his turn for the eyeball treatment: 'That would be weak!' Very fierce!

*My God! she's tough! Somehow he kept a straight face
as well!'*

~

Some more emails to the girls:

…*'I went out today looking for a walker for Mum - not sure
what prompted this but she has asked for it (she remembered the one
I rented for her late last year, which she flatly refused to use then.
That was three months ago!) Yesterday she told me it was 'good
when I had that thing to hold onto', so I've bought her one now - or
rather I used her money - not that she knows this. I've told yet
another lie and assured her the 'government' has loaned it to her.*

*She tried it out, wheeled it onto the verandah and there it's
stayed. The disconcerting thing is that she's taken to sitting on it,
just gazing out the window - without the brake on, of course -
with the potential of it scooting backwards and dumping her on
the floor. I've tried to explain about the brake and suggested her
favourite chair might be more comfortable but this is a novelty;
she's quite impressed with it.'*

March 2008:

*'Mum decided to make biscuits so I weighed everything for
her and set her up - have just finally put them in the oven. She's
forgotten most of the process but can still chant the recipe out and
direct me in the weighing, using the butter pat cut into chunks
for the weights. Also, of course, the paper must go in the oven
under the tray.*

*While she seems to accept that she needs me to do the
weighing she takes over for the kneading on the marble slab. I am*

allowed to grease the tin but she insists on pressing the mixture in (very unevenly - always managing to leave it about four cms thick one end and barely covering the bottom at the other.) There are ructions if I offer to do that.

Once in the oven, she leaves, so I can whip it out and re-spread the mix without her seeing. At least for once she chose a convenient time. Usually she announces she wants to cook just as I'm going out somewhere.

She was up at about three this morning. By the time I realised, she was out on the verandah and eating her toast! She insisted on finishing it so I waited, then I encouraged getting back into her nightie before going back to bed. She was all for climbing in with jumper etc. on - was quite crotchety. I finally left, turning off the light, calling out (as sweetly as I could with teeth grinding,)

'Good Night.'

'Good riddance!' came back out of the darkness!

This morning she was most confused - thought she'd slept in too late (though she still emerged around 7.30.) I decided not to notice whether she had breakfast again or not. She's currently out on the verandah having a cup of tea, which she ASKED ME to make - signs of deterioration. That's happening more and more.'

～

A month later, in April, Mum had another quite serious fall. As she climbed the stairs on her way up after her now-customary evening visit she fell backwards from about half-way up - flat on her back. I heard the clonk as her head hit the concrete. I raced out, fearing the worst and found her prone with blood pouring from the back of her head. (It's amazing how the scalp can bleed!)

There I was, trying to check her, fully expecting something HAD to have broken this time. But she was quite lucid, wanting to know if she'd broken the cup she was carrying - which I'd tried to take off her so she could use two hands on the railings but, as usual, she'd stubbornly insisted on carrying it herself.

After feeling her all over, waiting for a yelp, which never came, I finally asked her to gently try to move her arms and legs. Kneeling next to her, as she lay on her back, I was bending forward. Suddenly, up went all four limbs - straight into the air pointing at the sky - she nearly slugged me with one fist.

After a time I got her inside. Since she was walking normally, I decided she didn't need an ambulance - going to emergency would be an ordeal all of its own - one I really wanted to avoid. When I rang Richard to report the situation he left the decision with me.

It was only a small cut - about two cm. but about as deep as it could go in that spot (the middle of the back of the skull.) I disinfected and bandaged it as best I could and next day we saw a locum doctor, who serri-stripped it together and put a pressure pad and tighter bandage around the whole head. The bandage was to stay on for about a week 'til Bill Wilson could come to check it.

I wrote to the girls: *'Am keeping a very close eye on her, sleeping on a mattress on the floor outside her door (which she doesn't know about - I only bring it out after she's asleep.)*

Had quite a session with her last night going to bed. She

hasn't complained of a headache or any pain except for direct touch but last night when she was going to bed I, once again, tried to give her a couple of painkillers. This was after I'd had to deal with her patrolling round and round the house trying to sort things and make new piles of the clothes she drapes everywhere. Kept seeing something on the floor and bending over to pick it up then staggering sideways as she lost her balance!

I was pretty tired by this time and really didn't want to cope any more so, after the refusal of the Panadol I gave up and left. She got out of bed and slammed her door!

About an hour later I was ready for bed on my mattress so I opened the door to check her. Out she came, 'Why am I in so much pain? Am I being punished for something?'

I had to quickly shepherd her back into her room so she wouldn't see the mattress.

She'd removed the bandage and was just generally, incredibly indignant. I had a great hassle sorting her out, re-bandaging etc., FINALLY getting her to take the Panadol and then explaining how she needed to sleep on her side (again.)

'But I prefer sleeping on my back.'

'Yes, but the back of your head has a cut and that's why it hurts.'

She wouldn't listen when I kept trying to explain that she was injured (which of course she denies.) She just kept telling me she was still in pain. 'Why? why?'

I kept assuring her it would soon start to go if she'd just lie down, 'Well - I hope so! Two minutes later: 'It's still hurting now!' (Ye gods!)

At last she settled and I flaked. The great thing was that she slept right through to 6 a.m. (I had expected to have to get up to

*her a few times like the night before.) It was great! Then we both
slept again 'til 8 a.m. I feel a lot better today!*

*She was incredibly alert all day yesterday - didn't doze off
once - which is unheard of these days. Presumably this is because
of some sort of system shock. She's settling back a bit today and is
dozing on the verandah as I type.'*

My big problem then was trying to stop her from going
down the stairs to my place - at least until she'd healed and
her system was a bit more settled - I felt she was too
unsteady and vulnerable. So I tied a bright orange sarong
across the top of the stairs, showed her and explained that it
was there to remind her not to go down - to call me if she
needed anything. I went over and over it.

'Yes,' she agreed - 'that's sensible.'

I spent most of each day up with her, watching in case of
any change. One evening, at around six I left her, saying I
was just going down to feed Banjo and organise my meal.
The phone rang - I answered it on the downstairs extension
- and next minute, there she was outside my door!

'Did you hear the phone ringing?'

I hassled her back up; 'Didn't you remember? We tied
this here to remind you NOT to go downstairs? Just call out
to me!'

'No - you put it there to remind me to be careful!'

As I wrote in an email:

*'Visualise it: the sarong was still in place strung across like a
curtain between the two posts at the top. To go down she had
ducked under it - right at the top of the stairs!!! The mind
boggles!*

She's just lucky she didn't fetch up on the edge of a pot the other night and break her neck. Doesn't bear thinking about, really.'

I removed the sarong. I also removed all of the pot-plants from the landing and replaced them with an old foam mattress segment.

I continued to spend most of my time upstairs, working on my computer in the spare room, with one ear cocked, ready to head her off at the back door when she went looking for me.

Major arguments ensued.

I wrote in frustration;

'She still gets really exasperated about any fuss and trying to direct her or assist in any way with anything is still a major battle - it's so stressful for me.

But - dementia is quite fascinating! How can she be off the planet most of the time but still hold onto the stubbornness? Maybe that's a form of control.

I finally had to give up, keep away and revert to my most scientific strategy - keeping my fingers crossed!

So I'm not sure what's going to take Mum off this earth - or, the gods help me - when! She's so tough! Am still at the dreaming stage re travelling. One day?!

Last week I went to the huge annual Recreational Vehicle Show; still dreaming of perhaps buying that motorhome.

Yesterday I was talking to my friend, Lynn, about my dream - touring in my mythical motorhome. I said - 'If she doesn't die soon I'm going to have to take her with me!'

Lynn suggested that would be a good title for a book!

I have this feeling that she'll go on way past 100 and I'll be getting into my own dotage!'

Several days later: *'Yes - it makes NO difference to me when you phone - I am here every night - haven't thought about going out at night for many, many moons. I'll have totally got out of the habit by the time I'm free again! I must admit I think I've gone a bit stir crazy this past week - I truly dread the thought that Mum might become incapacitated or lingeringly ill. Being around each other constantly is damned difficult.*

Thank heavens her head is healing well - her system is in top shape.'

For the next week Mum slept later than usual and was too disoriented to manage her own breakfast. I wondered if we were entering a new era, where she would need more care. But eight days later, the morning after Dr. Bill removed the dressing, I found her up and preparing her grapefruit and cereal soon after seven.

I heaved a sigh of relief. It had been a trying week. I'd had to give up trying to prevent her from using the stairs. It just caused too much grief - for both of us!

Each evening, despite me going up and down very regularly during her meal preparation and repeating and repeating, 'No, there's no-one else coming for dinner, it's just veges for ONE - YOU!' and showing her, yet again, which switch turns the hotplate on etc. etc., she still trotted down at least three times.

I would walk behind her going up and she objected to that, but I gave up trying to head her off going down.

During that long week I wrote: *'My fingers are getting cramped! I tell you - I'm so glad I set up the separate living space (I KNEW it was important; now I REALLY know!) I reckon one of us would be dead by now - and it'd be me - if I'd had to live in the same house as her.*

She daily threatens to, 'Go back home if we're not going to be able to get along', always caused, of course, by her agitation and my ham-fisted attempts to sort it; why do I keep trying????

Thank the gods, although the dementia causes the frustrations, it helps her forget the friction quickly and we have civil exchanges most of the time. Pre-dementia, as you know, we would still have had conflict but she would have maintained the coldness endlessly. Small mercies. This IS better!

There! It's good to vent!'

~

Mum's 99th birthday was Monday, June 9th., 2008. Richard and Soe drove up from Canberra for the weekend, so we brought the celebration forward.

I invited my two cousins and their husbands to lunch on Saturday and we had a delightful celebration. Although she had previously always strenuously objected to having her photo taken, she had mellowed considerably regarding this and actually enjoyed the fuss, posing for photographs as she cut her cake, blowing out the two big candles and generally loving the novelty of being in a social group.

Inevitably, she was somewhat discombobulated by the time evening came. We had a garbled argument about her having a car that she lets me drive, wanting to be driven 'home now'. She became very shirty with me over it all.

'How can you say that you don't drive my car? What's wrong with you? Just take me home - now!'

I handed her over to Richard and Soe to try to sort it out and left. She always listened to whatever Soe suggested and never argued with her.

She slept in 'til almost 9 o'clock next morning and - amazingly! - wasn't upset about the time when she discovered how late it was. I guess she was diverted by their departure soon after late breakfast.

I wrote to Kriket:

'They've gone back to Canberra. No doubt I'll have a session with her this evening about cooking for a cast of thousands! We'll see.

So, even though tomorrow is officially the birthday, I'm not going to bother to tell her. She's already had an extended celebration - and forgotten it – so there's no point. If I mention it, she'll naturally expect something to happen and I simply don't have the energy.'

2 days later:

'Richard and Soe phoned in the morning but I asked them not to wish her 'Happy Birthday'. That was O.K. - they agreed. Mum happily took over the phone but the conversation became very garbled because they reminded her about being here on a visit and giving her a new jumper. All news to her of course!

She valiantly held up her end, obviously not having the slightest memory of any of it but was very gracious toward them. (It never ceases to amaze me how well she can 'wing it!') After we hung up I fetched the jumper and showed it to her.

'I've never seen this before - it's not mine'. Then, after a bit of thought: 'I didn't realise it was Christmas. You should have told me – I need to buy presents - what am I giving to everyone?' And so it went …

For the next hour, while I was working on photographs on the computer, she worried and worried over it, poor thing. She kept coming in, still carrying the jumper: 'Now… if it's Christmas, what are we going to feed them? When are they coming?' I'd explain – not Christmas – 'it was your birthday' and she'd wander off, still puzzling. Ten minutes later, in she'd come and we'd go through it all again. FINALLY, after going away for the fourth time she came in and announced - 'I've just worked it out! It was MY birthday wasn't it?' (YEEEESSSSSS!) Then:'99? That's ridiculous! How can that be? That can't be right.'

And so the day proceeded quietly until about six in the evening when Robbie and Chris from across the road arrived with their three daughters bringing a lovely bunch of flowers and small gifts. (Oh no! I thought - not at this time of night, please!) We so rarely actually have upstairs visitors - especially in the evening.

What with Mum's confusion, being totally overwhelmed and embarrassed by the attention (not having a clue who they were - or why they were there giving her presents but charmingly bluffing as though she totally did know) the dogs getting excited and Jade (a very shy, neurotic toy poodle I'm minding for three months) doing her usual skittering around hiding and peeping out from behind chairs and doors - chaos reigned!

Of course the little girls fell in love with Jade so I brought her out for some ooohs and ahhhs and cuddles, which she is slowly learning aren't entirely all bad things but she doesn't stop quivering.

Being right around the magic age of turning ten - that first oh-so-important double numbers birthday - the twins pointed out this is Mum's LAST double numbers birthday! Pretty impressive! I hadn't thought of that! Mum was delighted to learn she had turned 99 – it was complete news to her. (We'd only discussed it at least six times during the day!)

After they left I had great unravelling once again. Then soon after I went downstairs, Katy dropped in to visit Jade. She's Jade's owner's daughter and lives just across the park.

Mum came down while she was there and of course, thought she was one of the previous visitors so she tried to continue that interaction (which totally confused Katy.) THAT took a bit of sorting. Shades of a French Farce!

So the birthday has been DONE! Thank God!'

~

June brought a spate of serious night rambling -up to three times a night - between midnight and five a.m. Mum would get herself up, dress and make breakfast or have a bath or just wander around, turning all the lights on and rear-ranging the clothes draped on the lounge chairs.

Her progress in this wandering tended to depend on my state of exhaustion and how long it took me to register the tell-tale sounds. After four nights in a row I found myself becoming very 'ratty' one way and another.

One night around 1.30 a.m. there I was, shivering, in the bathroom begging her to get out of the bath and go back to bed, while she grumbled away at me and continued to vaguely splash water over her upper half ordering me to leave her alone.

I couldn't do that, despite her assuring me she would go back to bed. I knew full well that she would forget and proceed to try to get dressed etc. and I'd only have to drag myself out again. The previous night she'd started getting dressed three times - kept going back to bed, then half an hour later, it'd all be repeated.

I wrote:

'In the end I lost it and pulled the plug out. My patience is seriously limited at such times I have to admit! She stubbornly sat there until the bath was entirely empty - visibly furious - then she took forever to dry herself, carefully drying between every toe, patting herself over and over with the towel.

I finally got her back under the covers and thank the gods she slept right through. (Nothing like a warm bath, they say!)

It's getting hard.'

Thank heavens it wasn't always that intense, averaging just three to four times a week. However, I realised the anticipation on the 'off' nights was also beginning to take a toll on me.

~

That was when I installed a baby monitor, hiding the microphone under her bed. That way I could hear her when she first stirred to go to the bathroom - and returned – or not. If silence ensued, I knew I needed to get upstairs fast.

It meant more interruptions to my sleep but I didn't always have to get up and the time dealing with it was reduced because I usually could deflect her before she was into some activity. On the way through the kitchen I'd fill the jug so I could re-fill her hot water bottles - they could be an enticement.

In July I wrote:

'Sometimes in the cold wee hours, she is even apologetic about disturbing me but most often she gets really indignant.

'If it's not the right time to be getting up, what are you doing here then?'

I have now spoken to her doctor and have permission to get her to take a full sleeping tablet instead of half when there is a series of interrupted nights (Boy! I can totally sympathise with resorting to sedation under some circumstances!)

It's intriguing that she has begun this at the very coldest time of the year! She agrees that bed is more comfortable and that, yes, she is cold (paddling around bare foot in a light nightdress.) How she avoids catching something serious I fail to understand. It's not natural!

Yes, of course, I've tried to put long underwear on her before going to bed - or even winter pyjamas - but she's still seriously STUBBORN. 'THIS is what I wear to bed!' flapping an ancient, threadbare nightie at me.

As an attempted antidote, I've been taking her on 'route marches' every afternoon lately - a short walk at about 4.30 p.m. to try to tire her out a bit and get bracing air into her lungs and (touch wood) we've gone through four nights in a row, when she hasn't wandered! She slept 'til 9 a.m this morning!

Dare I hope? But there's no anticipating! Probably just luck and tonight will be a different story. Never mind - I can cope!'

Despite the increasing need for me to be around most of the time, I was very fortunate that I was sometimes still able to go out during the day for a few hours, leaving Mum in the house. I was always grateful that she never attempted to wander anywhere during daylight hours. I absolutely dreaded the thought that I'd possibly have to lock doors when she was awake. I just couldn't have done it. And as long as I limited the absence, she coped on her own very well.

Even a brief change of scenery was rejuvenating for me.

$$\sim$$

The first week of July, Karin, my older daughter, husband, Micheal and seven-year-old grand-daughter, Jasmine, flew down from Queensland for eight days, which was wonderful, though of course it threw Mum 'out' somewhat.

However, interestingly, the night wandering wasn't too bad at all while they were there. Perhaps the novelty of interacting with other people all day tired her out more. There was no way of knowing when she would wander - I never did learn the triggers.

She just loved having the family there. I remember one evening we all had dinner down in my place and afterwards there was a competition to touch our toes without bending knees. I knew Mum could still do this with ease - she practiced often - but the family was mightily impressed! We even took her on a picnic to West Head one day.

Matt was down for the weekend as well and the family was delighted to have an outing with her after years of her not really wanting to participate in anything. Despite my misgivings about the impact of such a novel situation, I encouraged it. It meant I could go as well.

The idea was to keep the jaunt as short as possible, allowing for the drive and a picnic lunch. She loved it all, commenting on the scenery and the view, tucking into the picnic and happily chatting to everyone. We had a great day.

However the inevitable consequence came with a vengeance … We returned in time for afternoon tea (always a necessity) but the outing was rather more than her mind could cope with.

At about 4.30, I drove off to shop for food and while I was gone she began preparing for bed, rejecting all Karin's protestations that it wasn't yet time.

I'd warned the family not to let Mum know I was her daughter but in the confusion Karin's 'Just wait until Helen comes home' brought an unexpected rejoinder.

'Helen is MY daughter and I know what she wants better than you!'

However, when I returned I immediately became 'her' again.

Mum had her habits well established. Her schedule seemed to be indelibly printed onto her sub-conscious, always going by the time on the clock - a skill she never lost. But that day even a suggestion from Karin that we hadn't had dinner, that she check the time (often a 'stranger' would prompt some respect and politeness) and reminding her about Matthew being here (one of the four people she never forgot) plus other reasonable entreaties, simply exacerbated the situation. She was beyond connection.

When I arrived back half an hour later she was positively bristling - very indignant, disturbed and angry.

I had foolishly left the key in the back door when we arrived home and things became more complicated when I discovered Mum had managed to lock it then immediately misplace the key. The long-relinquished habit in preparation for bed had returned. (I eventually found it in the oven.)

Finally, at 5.15 she stomped off to her bed without dinner. Anticipating a very disrupted night, gauging she'd probably start wandering around midnight, I made sure I went off early to try to get as much sleep as I could. However, she was obviously exhausted and slept all the way through to 8.30 next morning.

From then on outings were limited to the occasional, well-timed, gentle drive down to the lake to sit and watch the ducks!

We had one other hilarious evening together. Micheal is an avid sports fan and the State of Origin was on that night. My paltry little T.V. set downstairs was just not acceptable so I suggested we all watch it upstairs with Mum on her large set. The problem was, Mum disliked sport of any kind.

In his retirement my dear father, a lifelong follower of rugby, had been relegated to the spare room to watch his precious sport on a tiny black and white T.V.

I explained to Mum that this was a very important match and, being hostess, she graciously agreed. She was most amused when my family appeared in their maroon gear - scarves, flags etc.

Then it began. At the first tackle Mum leapt up in horror! 'Goodness, it's so rough! Why are they doing that?' Then she'd pat Micheal on the arm: 'You don't do those things do you?'

This continued for the entire game.

Amazingly, she stayed the course - ever the hostess - no doubt hating every minute of it but providing high entertainment for all of us with her indignant running commentary but joining in to clap (in bewilderment) when we roared over every try.

Between constantly explaining it to her and the excitement of a win, a good time was had by all.

I was so happy to have had part of my family there - for myself as well as Mum. Even though she didn't remember the visit afterwards, she loved it all at the time, specially meeting her great-grand-daughter.

Such moments are so precious.

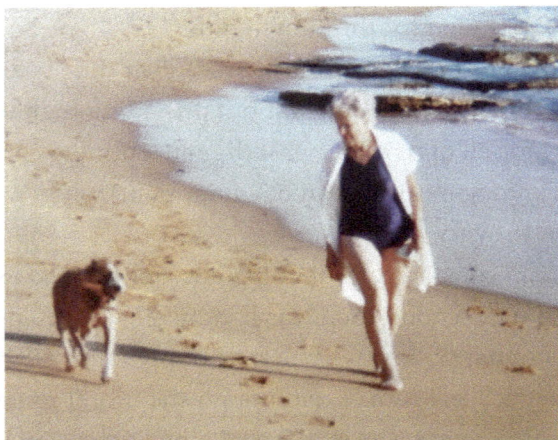

Aged 94, morning swim with ' Podge' and below, on
the back steps with Banjo.

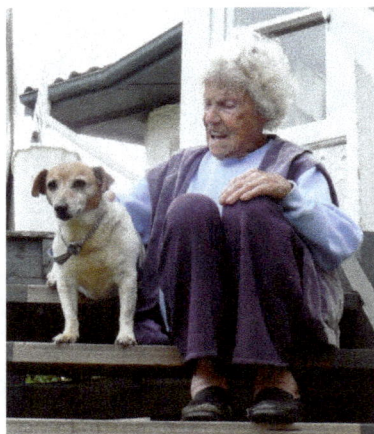

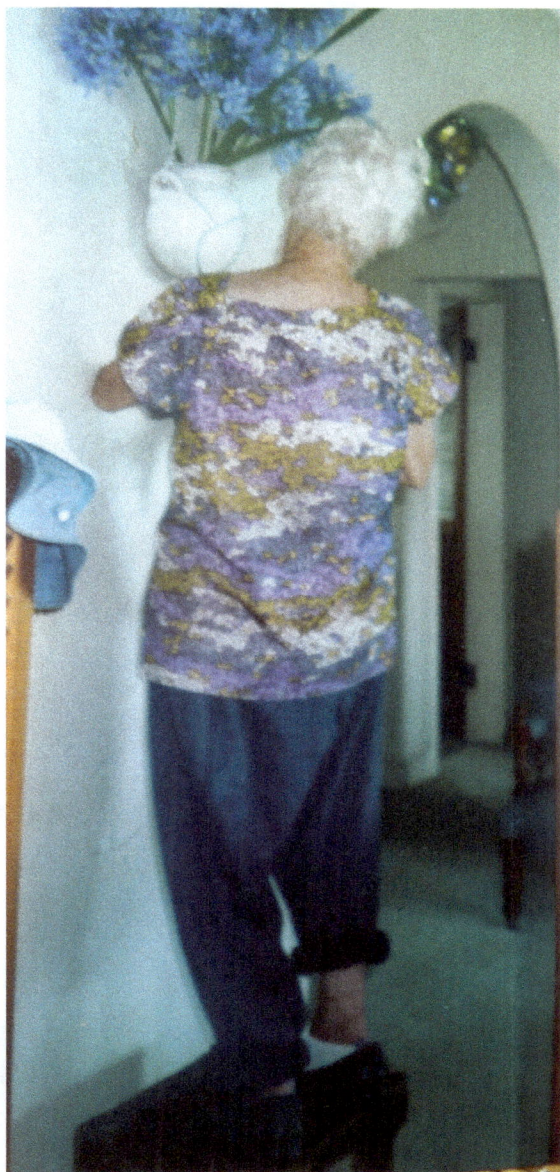

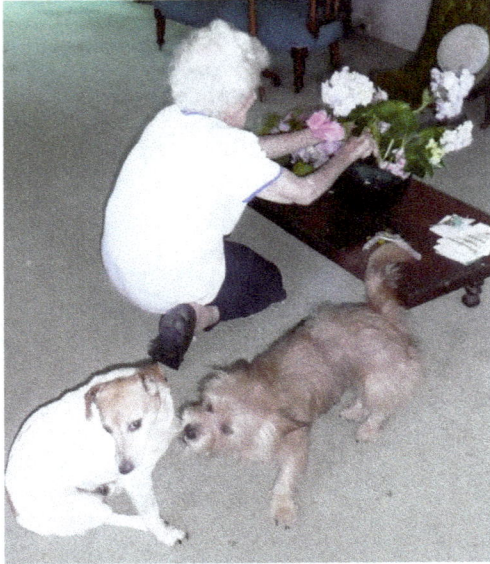

Previous page and above: Favorite past-time
- arranging flowers. I finally had to remove
that stool so she couldn't climb up. Over
page: No job was too hard … but sometimes
it was good to just sit back and relax.

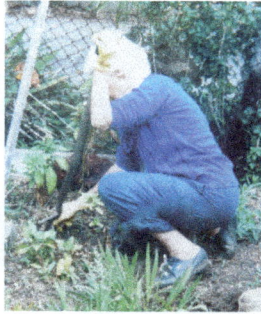
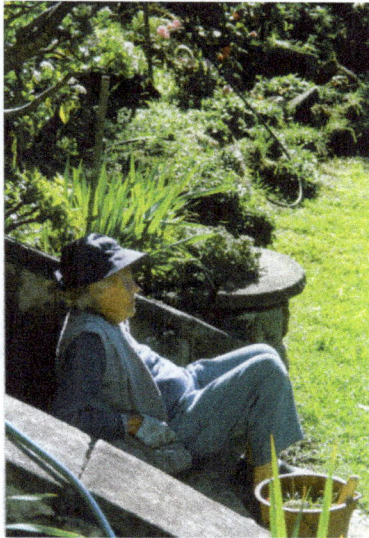

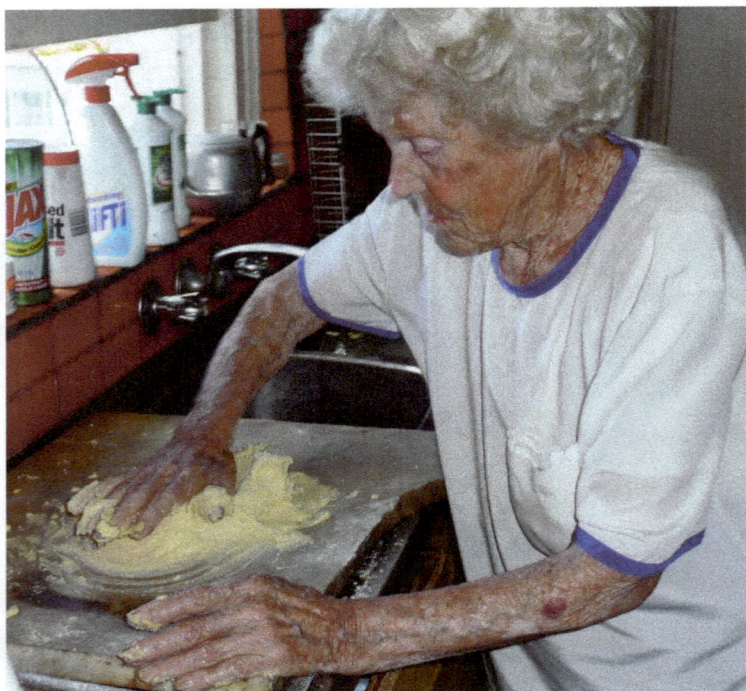

'You must knead the shortbread dough on a marble slab.' Edna made her last batch the week before her accident - at 99. Over page: Favorite place

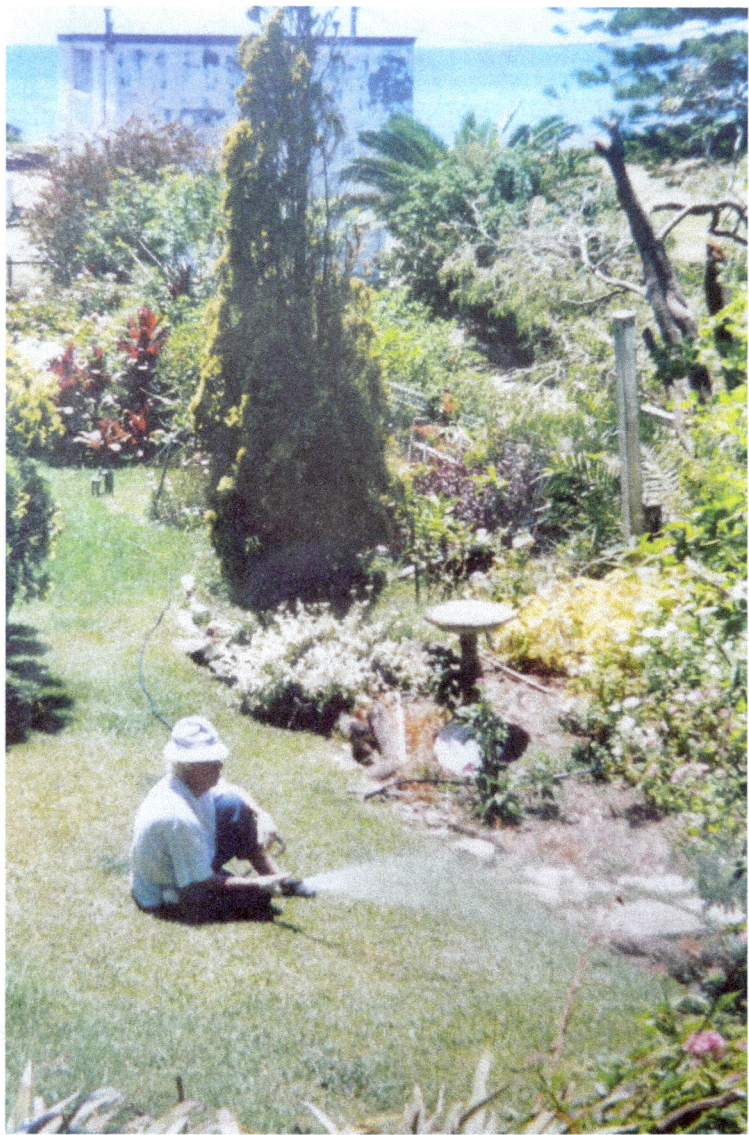

'Failure is a unique method of being granted another chance to get it right.' - Unknown

PART THREE

As July 2008 passed, once the family had left, we resumed the 'normal' routines. I was still able to get down to the beach for a short swim each morning. Plus I kept up Mum's afternoon walks. In fact the days were relatively quiet because Mum dozed so much, making up for all the lost sleep during the night.

Unfortunately, I didn't have that luxury and was more and more aware that I was being stretched - not beyond endurance - but definitely on the way.

My friend Lynn's husband had recently been moved to a nursing home causing great grief for her, which I could identify with. Our regular phone-calls increased. I can't emphasise enough how important this contact was, being able to share our comparable situations and vent without any constraint.

My greatest fear was that I would reach a stage where I felt I couldn't cope any longer, which would mean Mum would have to be placed into High Care. I dreaded the thought. The locked doors, the regimentation, would be pure torture for her. I was determined to avoid this at all costs.

~

Back before Christmas I had applied to ACAT (the Aged Care Assessment Team) to have her officially assessed. It was important to be prepared for her to be taken into temporary care if an emergency arose to take me out of action for any reason.

At last, in May, after seven months on the waiting list, ACAT made an appointment to come to the house for the assessment.

I phoned the co-ordinator and explained that it would be best if I had the meeting with the assessor, an occupational therapist, rather than involve Mum but - no - Mum was the client and she must be interviewed personally. I warned her that Mum was not capable of providing lucid or correct information and requested a booking for a follow-up interview. This was also refused.

We sat around the dining room table, me opposite the assessor and Mum between us, happily making small talk, switching to her customary 'hostess' mode. Out came the clipboard and the questions began:

'Do you live here on your own, Edna?'

'Yes, of course.'

'You've got a lovely garden - who helps you with that?'

'Goodness, I do the gardening - I've always had gardens. I don't need help with that!'

'Do you do your own shopping?'

'Oh! Yes. I catch the bus every week.'

This is a minuscule example of the farce we endured for the next hour or so, while Mum spun the most amazing stories about all her gardening and cooking etc. with me surreptitiously gesturing 'No! No!' and the assessor totally ignoring me, being completely taken in.

She focussed entirely on her client, sailing through her form, ticking boxes against questions I couldn't see upside down, not bothering to even ask them. I knew her assumptions were all wrong. Mum rallied unbelievably - sounded completely lucid, independent and extraordinarily convincing.

Although I knew Mum would unravel as soon as it was over and I'd need to do a lot of explaining, I left her and followed the 'expert' out to her car:

'Most of what my mother told you was quite incorrect. I explained to the woman in your office that she has advanced dementia. We need to make a time to straighten this out.'

She just brushed me off, telling me she was satisfied with the interview - that she had to move on to another appointment.

I had been told by my carer friends how they had been ignored by medicos and other professionals when their loved one was in hospital or being interviewed by authorities like ACAT.

Unbelievable! We are the ones who live with the situation - we are undoubtedly the experts on our particular individual.

I was furious but, of course, had to move back inside to work through the aftermath - Mum's inevitable confusion. Having an official person come to interview her was very impressive and she was full of questions.

I fabricated some story about a government survey of elderly people still living in their own homes, which she nodded knowingly over. Her mind had risen valiantly to the occasion but once over, it descended into a whirling maelstrom.

My followup phone-call to ACAT next morning, trying to clarify and correct the answers was greeted with a brisk: 'The report with our recommendations will be sent to you in due course.'

It arrived almost three months later - in late July - just after the family's visit, identifying Mum as low-care (as I suspected) with ticks in the Cognition boxes against questions she hadn't even bothered to put to Mum. It was almost laughable but desperately serious from my point of view. This report was the basis for emergency placement for Mum. The result of housing her in a low care facility, even for a short period, would potentially be disastrous.

After several attempts at demanding another interview - for myself only - which was always refused, I redid the questionnaire/report - correcting it with red pen - and returned it with a terse letter. Eventually I received a reply making an appointment for late September - two months hence.

We soldiered on.

I also consulted with Richard, pointing out that I was going to need to have someone available to move in for short respite periods. I had enquired about professional services and discovered the costs were exorbitant. However, through the Carer Support Group I managed to find a lovely woman, Ann, who did relatively reasonably-priced, private, live-in respite.

In order to familiarise Ann with Mum's routines and needs, I initially employed her for two short stints every week. I also wanted Mum to become used to her and (hopefully) even remember her. Whether she did or not was actually irrelevant - she simply enjoyed the diversion.

Sleeping. At night. There had to be a way. A referral to a gerontologist was arranged for August. A new sleeping tablet prescription obtained.

This followup letter, written at the beginning of September to the specialist describes the result of that:

'Dear Dr. Parker,

You recently changed my Mum's sleeping tablets from Alladorm to Temazapam. You suggested I let you know how they are going.

We have tried them now for almost two weeks and, while it is really easy to give her a whole tablet, because they are so small, I feel they aren't strong enough for her. A couple of times when she's been particularly disoriented in the evening, she is able to stay up without becoming drowsy for as long as an hour and a half after taking one.

Normally I give her the tablet half an hour before she's preparing for bed - at around 8.30. She still often wakes several times a night, starting any time from 12.30 a.m., then wandering, getting dressed etc. and appearing quite alert.

Usually I do manage to get her back to bed without too much trouble and she does finally go back to sleep but it has something of an impact on me, because I can't always get back to sleep so easily.

This morning was a slightly new story. At 3 a.m. I found her wandering, with all the lights in the house on and when I asked her to go back to bed she became very agitated and actually violent, trying to hit and punch me.(She's amazingly strong and I had to hold her off quite firmly.)

She began shouting out 'Help' and 'Go away' at the top of her voice and even grabbed at a glass of water on her side table to try to throw at me. It took a huge effort to calm her enough for me to be able to back away. Then she insisted on having lights on and staying awake, commanding me to help her get dressed, getting very angry.

She didn't recognise me, of course, but usually, when she becomes agitated and delusional, after I leave her for a short while she settles down. However, this morning, even when she was finally lying back in bed (but insisting on having the light on) and I left her for up to 15 minutes at a time, whenever I returned she again began screaming to 'Go away' at the top of her voice.

This is a new behaviour. After an hour she at last turned the light off and went back to sleep, going through until much later than her normal waking time.

While she is often much more argumentative at these times, feeling thwarted and indignant when I suggest she needs to go back to bed, this morning we plumbed new depths!

I've observed that she can be weirdly clear-headed at 3 or 4 a.m. This is when I'd really like her to stay sound asleep.

Could we try another sleeping aid please? Immediately? For the first time ever, I am planning (hoping?!) to bring in a live-in *carer so I can go away for a tiny break next week on September 8th & 9th.*

I have only been able to get away infrequently in the past and right now I'm very concerned about being able to do this next week. Obviously I need to feel confident that she is as settled as we could hope for someone else to care for her.

For me this is something of an emergency ...'

I didn't mention to Dr. Parker the days of mortification I suffered after that. Mum had bruises all over her forearms from when I restrained her as she tried to hit me with the glass.

Thank heaven for thick walls in brick houses! I can't imagine how the neighbours didn't hear the screams. I kept half-expecting the police to turn up as I sat out that long, cold hour in the dark outside her room, waiting for her to settle.

~

Yes! I had bitten the bullet! Several 'graduate' carer friends were planning a two-night stay in a guesthouse on the Central Coast and I planned to join them.

I was confident about Ann - had written up a schedule and copious notes for her. I'd introduced another sleeping tablet, which seemed more effective. I just had to sort out ACAT after I returned.

This was the beginning of a new era.

The same week I was dealing with the above, I had a back tooth extracted. The cavity developed into a fistula on my sinus, which potentially could mean an operation, so I was on antibiotics, in excruciating pain and generally pretty run down.

On 3rd. September my dentist sent me to a specialist - a most wonderful man, who responded to my no doubt somewhat incoherent description of my situation ending with: 'I CAN'T have an operation and I HAVE to be able to go away for two nights next week!'

I must have had an impact. He undertook to clean and dress the cavity daily to try to avoid the operation. Amazingly, for the next 5 days - even over the weekend! - he opened his office specially to be able to do it at seven a.m. every morning, allowing me to have my treatment and get home before Mum had properly surfaced. Thank the heavens - and this brilliant, caring man - the fistula receded. I had the last treatment the Monday morning of departure.

Ann arrived. I kissed Mum good-bye - drove away - collected my friends and was free! I took the precaution of driving my own car in case I had to return urgently.

Bliss! No demands for two whole days of relaxing with good company, intelligent conversation and food cooked by someone else, plus a chance to read in peace - not to mention two full nights' sleep - all without having to watch the clock!

On my return on Wednesday morning, feeling like I could handle anything again, I found a peaceful, serene mother, ensconced in her customary spot, suggesting a cup of tea.

I think she vaguely recognised me as the lady from downstairs but she was oblivious to the fact that I'd been away. Ann, the treasure, had managed beautifully and

Mum had totally behaved herself - no night wandering - and she hadn't even indulged in any secret Nan's business - or if she had she had successfully disposed of the evidence.

The future looked bright.

~

That night we went through our routine without many hiccups and at about 9.30 I crept back up to check on Mum before locking up. She was deeply asleep.

I'd learned not to go to bed straight away - if she woke she used to go out to the verandah window just above my door and call out to me, so I gave it another half hour.

All was quiet. I jumped into the shower.

Just as I emerged I heard her voice - quite strident. Obviously she'd been calling and I hadn't heard over the noise of the water.

On went a sarong - up the stairs - through the back door into the fully illuminated house. Into the bedroom. No Mum. Bathroom - the same. All rooms - no Mum.

My stomach began rising to my throat. Had she fallen behind a door or a curtain? I called and called.

Running. Frantic.

The doors were all still firmly closed.

But she was gone.

It felt completely surreal.

I'd looked out on the verandah first but went out again, calling, calling her name. Then I heard a faint voice through the window at the far end.

I suddenly realised my grandfather's heavy wooden

chest full of rusty old tools - a fixture that had sat under a window half-way along the verandah for forty years - too heavy for me to remove - was now under that window.

The window was open ...

'Ah no! Please No!' My heart leapt into my throat.

I looked out and there she was on the concrete path below, in the dark, curled on her side.

Somehow I got through the kitchen, down the stairs and around to the other side of the house, mind rushing, every nerve-end tingling. Trying to prepare ... for what?

I crouched over her - she was alive - moving. I dashed back the few metres into my room, grabbed a pillow, a blanket and torch.

It had begun to drizzle.

When I rejoined her she was trying to get up and asking where she was.

'You've fallen out of the window - you climbed on the box! Please! You mustn't move.' I had to shout to make her hear me and I was incapable of being remotely calm.

'I thought you couldn't hear me. ... Am I in the garden? ... Oh! I did a silly thing!'

Unbelievably, she actually realised for a fleeting moment what had happened.

Apparently, when she called from her usual window and I didn't respond immediately, she decided she needed to lean out further from a different window - hence the box to give her extra height.

She had toppled three metres down onto the concrete path.

Experience had taught me that shock wasn't terribly likely
to occur but I felt sure she must have injured herself terribly
and expected pain to engulf her any second. But, no! She
began to try to struggle onto her hands and knees; I restrained
her and begged her to lie still on the pillow while I proceeded
very carefully to handle her all over, moving limbs, feeling
her arms and legs, gently feeling down her back, both of us
getting wetter as the sprinkle began to intensify.

She kept insisting that she wasn't in pain and she wasn't
staying out in the rain.

'I want to go inside!' It was a command.

I was equally determined that she shouldn't move,
although I was beginning to dare to imagine that, miracu-
lously, she wasn't too badly injured.

'If you won't help me I'll crawl, then.' Pushing at me she
tried to roll over again.

My brain was tumbling. She might be in control but I
was trembling all over. We were shouting at each other.

The rain was increasing. Nothing I said, trying to
explain how serious it was, made any difference to her. She
became angrier and angrier. Her iron will completely
took over.

I gathered my thoughts. It was only about four metres to
the door of my room. I'd had two previous experiences
when she'd been unaffected by what should have been seriously damaging falls, both involving concrete.

Although quite small, she was too heavy for me to lift so
I tried to roll her onto the blanket, thinking I could drag her
along on that but I couldn't get any co-operation. Half-

sitting, she flailed at me with her hands, arms wheeling. She refused to lie down again.

I remembered the walker upstairs. Time for drastic action. I yelled at her to stay still, promising I'd help her inside - flew up and back in record time. Heart thumping, praying to every kind spirit in the universe, I sat on the walker and as carefully as I could I cradled her under the arms and slid her onto my lap, supporting her body with my legs, then slowly paddled backwards with my feet 'til we got to the door.

She groaned when I lifted her and I inwardly cringed at the thought of the damage I was inflicting but desperation ruled. I shut my mind to all the dire possibilities and at last managed to roll us both sideways onto the bed next to the door.

No question this time - she had to go to hospital.

Mercifully the ambulance responded really quickly. The paramedics went into action - so professional and reassuring - cutting her clothes away, putting her into a brace and securing her onto a stretcher.

When I told them what had happened they exchanged a look. While one efficiently attended to Mum, who was talking, though very garbled, his partner requested that I show him the window and the spot where she'd fallen. The soaked pillow and blanket were in a jumble on the path. I took him upstairs and showed him how the box had been dragged along the verandah - there were scrape marks.

I was distraught but it began to penetrate my brain that they would very reasonably suspect violence on my part. I went into an explanation about why she was locked in. I kept telling him my mother had dementia but was abnormally tough - and very strong-willed. Yes, I hated myself but I really felt I had no alternative but to relocate her once I thought she was still pretty much in one piece. His skepticism and disapproval were palpable.

A second ambulance was called. I threw on some clothes, grabbed my bag and climbed into the front next to the driver. Off we went, sirens blaring, the front vehicle forging through to clear a way as we raced to Royal North Shore Hospital, 40 minutes away.

The paramedic in the back with Mum settled her and re-checked all her vital signs, which he reported were good. Then, as we sped through red lights and past stationary vehicles he picked up a clipboard and began taking details.

'Name? … Date of birth?

'Ninth of June 1909'.

Dead silence as they did the maths.

'Holy Christ!' This expletive from the driver, glancing at me sideways, 'She's 99?'

It was close to midnight when she was taken into emergency and - bless them, tended to immediately. The paramedics made their report, repeating my story of the fall from a window onto concrete, with me hovering, staying as close to Mum's head as I could, trying to reassure her, but thinking, as I listened, how truly unbelievable the story was. I'd gone through the dreadful experience but it didn't sound likely - even to me.

She never lost consciousness but her mind was unable to comprehend, so she went into a sort of limbo. I held her hand, desperate to somehow shield her.

The decision was made to take her for multiple scans and x-rays and I crawled onto a chair in the waiting room wishing I was a praying person, cursing myself for daring to move her, trying to prepare for the worst.

Someone came to fill out another form. I managed to drink a cup of tea; explained about the advanced dementia. I begged them not to try to ask her any questions - to please come to me. And PLEASE DON'T operate or attempt to resuscitate.

I recalled stories from other carers about how medicos insisted on drastic treatment or resuscitation. An elderly carer friend, who had been away with us, told us about his dearly loved wife, in her eighties, who had lost the power of speech and become bed-ridden. He had cared for her for many years and when she developed pneumonia, he saw it as a blessing. However, despite his requests, the Doctor brought her through it and he had spent the last months sitting by her bed, watching her struggle, requiring assistance with eating, toileting and every other personal need.

I was trying to gear up for a confrontation but - bless them again - they showed nothing but amazing under-standing and sympathy.

Hours later they returned her, without the brace, the only detectable injury a slight crack in the front of her pelvis, presumably caused when she toppled forward over the windowsill. Unbelievably, I was told that this would heal itself with bed-rest.

Everyone just kept shaking their heads. It didn't seem possible. Admiring whispers of '99!' were exchanged as we ascended in the lift to the secure ward. By then Mum was dozing.

The efficient emergency staff had supplied the ward with all the information - I didn't have to go over everything again - a massive relief. The adrenaline rush had subsided and I was thoroughly exhausted. I managed to get some sleep in the chair next to her bed.

In the morning she was awake and talking, asking where she was, why she was there, when was she going home? But she didn't want to get up - she had bad bruising down her back and any movement caused her pain, which they efficiently and mercifully covered with morphine.

Richard and Soe drove to Sydney immediately and sat by her while I caught a cab home to change, collect personal items, feed and walk Banjo.

They stayed at the house and trekked over every day. I settled into a routine of spending each night at the hospital into the afternoon, then dashing home in the late afternoon for a couple of hours. I'd eat dinner and comfort my little bewildered Banjo, whose steady peaceful existence had been shattered, before returning for the night vigil. Matt arrived down from Coffs Harbour to lend support.

Over the next few days, the dementia proved a blessing, as she drifted into her own world.

We were just waiting.

Apart from the pain control, there was no treatment and we were told she could well recover, though they couldn't make predictions. We were also told that she couldn't stay in hospital for too many days so we discussed the logistics of taking her home and bringing nurses in if necessary.

I tried to blot out any thought of her not being able to eventually return home. I'd finally organised the lovely Ann, who, though costly, I could bring in, when necessary, to relieve me. I was all geared up, that very week, to straighten ACAT out and have her correctly assessed. I'd successfully stopped her leaving the house on her night wanders.

I finally felt I was truly on top of everything.

~

Mum dozed much of the time but, when awake, engaged in quite lively conversation - our usual aimless verbal wandering around diverse topics and lots of singing.

Various words would strike a song memory. For example, telling me she couldn't see very well any more diverted into 'My eyes are dim, I cannot see … ' at the top of her voice, with me joining in.

'I have not brought my specs with meeeee.'

'Daisy, Daisy' was popular, along with many other old evergreens, which we warbled through, to the amusement of the three other ladies in the ward.

One morning, suddenly, a soft dreamy expression came over her face. She began telling me about the boyfriend she'd had before my father. I'd heard about Mervyn in my childhood. They were very young. She was only about 18 when they met and he was a little older - apparently from 'the wrong side of the tracks' - a poor boy, who my grandfather disapproved of.

However, over a couple of years, they 'kept company'

meeting as often as they could and it was very serious. When the Great Depression hit he had to leave town looking for work and they never saw each other again. But she never forgot him.

Now she told me: 'A boy loved me once.' Her eyes were dreamy, gazing back mistily over 80 plus years.

'Really? Who was that?'

'His name was Mervyn and he loved me ... I loved him but Dad didn't think he was good enough. We had to meet secretly.'

'How lovely. What happened? Did he go away?'

'Ye-es ... ' She was a bit hesitant, so I changed the subject.

'Then you met Laurie and after a few years you married him.'

'Laurie? Yes, I married Laurie. He was a bank boy. Everyone wanted to marry a bank boy because they had superannuation. He thought I was nice... he loved me too.'

We agreed that Laurie was a lovely man; I almost got onto a sticky wicket there, because she wanted to know how I knew him but I managed to fob her off.

She drifted off again.

I freely admit that I was wishing for her to let go - to give up at last - but for the first two or three days she defied all expectations. However, she wasn't eating very much and on the fourth day the morphine was increased so that she slept more and more. Ever so gradually I watched my Mum gently moving away.

$\sim$

On the fifth morning, Sunday, she rallied when Richard and Soe, Robbie and her husband, Ian, visited. She knew them all and chatted happily for a short while. Then after they left, she sank into a deep peaceful sleep, while I read in the chair next to her.

At about 3 p.m. she suddenly woke and asked the customary 'Where am I?' By then her voice had become very childlike, the voice of a plaintive little girl. She was having no food but I had taken in fruit and I asked if she'd like some.

I was peeling grapes and slipping tiny portions between her lips, then squeezing mandarin segments so the juice could run onto her tongue. She literally lapped at it, asking, 'More please? Can I have some more? So sweet! mmmmmmm.'

Suddenly her eyes widened and, looking straight at me said in a pathetic, pleading voice; 'Is it a sin?'

I reassured her that it wasn't a sin; she could have as much as she liked. She'd close her eyes and I'd think she was asleep but then: 'More please?... Thank you! You're very kind.'

After a while, she became a little more alert: 'So kind ... Who ARE you?'

I felt my mother was dying - the conscious intervals were further and further apart. I became sentimental. Crossed my fingers. Perhaps she wouldn't hear.

'I'm your daughter, Helen,' I said quietly.

The eyes flew open: 'Who?' The voice stronger.

Damn! I'd done it again! I began mentally slapping myself.

With all my experience - how could I have succumbed?

O.K. - Diversion time. I hastily offered her a piece of grape. It was rejected. She was looking straight at me.

'WHO are you?'

I was bending over, quite close to her: 'I'm Helen, your daughter.' Her eyes stared straight into mine,

'My daughter - Helen? … You're NOT!'

Time to back-paddle: 'Well it's not important. Here I've got a delicious mandarin for you.'

But her mind had become sharper than it had been for many, many months. My proffered hand was brushed aside. There was not a hope of diverting her.

'What name did you say?'

'Helen.'

'Helen? … Yes! I DID have a daughter called Helen … but YOU'RE not her!'

'Well that's O.K.' I felt a new anguish. The days of vigil were beginning to tell. 'Why don't you have a little rest now?'

She'd used quite a bit of energy - been awake for about half an hour. I desperately wanted her to fade off again and she actually did seem to start to drift away. I watched her eyes beginning to droop, just as a baby's will slowly close, then half-open, then close again. I sat back thankfully.

False hope! Suddenly she was alert once more, staring right at me. I leaned forward.

The little child's voice had disappeared. My feisty mother was eyeballing me, totally alert:

'Are you telling me you're my daughter?'

'Er … Yes.'

The struggle for cognition was visible on her face. After days of mostly mumbling nonsense, now, incredibly, her mind had rallied and sharpened and she would not let this go. Minutes passed, then her face cleared.

'So, you've been away! Is that it? I haven't seen you for a long while?'

The time had come to be honest - no more fibs. After all, my foot was now firmly in 'it' and for all I knew this may be the last conversation I would have with my mother.

'No, actually, we've seen rather a lot of each other over the last little while.'

This was slowly digested, her eyes fixed on mine. Now the voice came firm and vibrant:

'Well! If that's the case - you haven't made much of an IMPRESSION on me!'

Hmmnnnn - both barrels! Why would I expect anything to be different? Somehow, I kept a straight face.

'Looks like I'm going to have to make more of an effort then, doesn't it?'

'You certainly ARE!' Her response came straight back, *very* loud - strident.

'O.K. Well, I definitely will, I promise. But, now that's settled, I think you must be feeling a bit tired, what about a little rest? I'll be right here.'

Nothing doing - now she was on a roll.

'Can you cook?' she demanded.

'Er, yes, what do you have in mind?' *How the hell can your crazy, addled mind suddenly be so sharp?*

'Can you make a tart?'

I used to make tarts, many long years ago. I knew my

mother was dying. No more untruths. 'Yes, I can make a tart. What flavour would you like?'

'Apricot! ... No! ... Chocolate!'

'Right! I'm going home soon to feed and walk the dog so I'll make you a chocolate tart and bring it back this evening.'

'Good! We'll eat it together.'

Finally, she was satisfied. She almost instantly slipped into a deep sleep.

I smiled to myself as I walked to my car - the body might, perhaps, be finally succumbing but that indomitable spirit was totally intact and I'd long since accepted that in my mother's opinion I'd never measure up!

I did lie - just that one last time. I didn't make a tart - I trusted that a lapse of two or three hours would take care of that memory and sure enough, when I returned, she had virtually lapsed into a coma.

Next morning the gerontologist told me it was just a matter of, possibly, hours and, not only did they agree to keep her in hospital, she was transferred into a private room.

She never woke properly again. The family visited but all through Monday and Tuesday she stayed in this state, just occasionally rallying slightly, always calling, 'Helen! Helen!' - clutching at the air.

Each time I squeezed her hand: 'Helen's here.' And she'd mumble, 'Helen's here', relax and slip away again.

These were the only times she'd used my name in almost two years. Amazing! The 'knowing' - the incredible capacity of the brain. Intriguingly, somewhere in her sub-conscious, as her life began to ebb, she identified a precious, comforting lifeline to cling to.

I stayed with her.

~

Some time after midnight on Wednesday morning, the beginning of the seventh day, her breathing began to falter, becoming slower and slower. She was lying on her back, with her head turned, facing me. I had a recliner chair right next to her and I moved over so I could lay my head on the pillow, our faces close.

We stayed that way, with me holding both her hands, lightly dozing, but aware of her breathing, which became more and more rasping as it slowed.

The interval between each breath stretched longer and longer.

As I lay there expecting each gasp to be her last, the eyes which had been closed for over 48 hours suddenly opened. Those light, forget-me-not blue, eyes I'd known all my life were staring into mine once again.

I suppose it's fanciful but I truly believe she had full awareness as we held each other's gaze. I moved closer, clasping her hands, my arm across her shoulder and we stayed that way, eyes locked, for probably ten minutes.I was murmuring to her to let herself go, telling her to fly, trying to reassure her it was alright, although I knew she couldn't hear me.

Her ragged breaths gently slowed, coming further and

further apart until, at last - silence - her eyes still fastened to mine. I think it was about 3 a.m.

At the grand age of 99 years and 99 days she was free.

I stayed lying next to her, holding her, weeping, yes, but relieved. And oh, so grateful! I was visualising her spirit having a wonderful adventure, clear-brained and happy, rushing to be with her sisters and mother, as we'd so often playfully discussed.

After some time I realised it probably had to be made official so I called the nurse. She summoned a doctor, who closed my mother's eyes and pronounced her deceased.

They kindly assured me I could stay with her for as long as I wanted - to let the desk know when I was ready to leave.

I saw no point in rousing Richard and Soe. It was almost morning and that would be time enough.

After probably another hour I began to gather my thoughts. I was fairly exhausted and, with peak hour due soon, I would have to negotiate heavy Sydney traffic to drive home. I needed to leave well before then so I said my last, loving farewell to my Mum and went to the desk.

Being the secure ward, the only way out was to ask the staff to release the locked door. I'd been through it many times over the past week.

The nurse on duty asked me to wait: I presumed I needed to fill out a form or sign something. Although, I didn't quite understand because we'd had the discussion about her brain donation and that was all in hand. These things are beautifully organised, I'd discovered. There isn't the great urgency in removing a brain as there is for other organs. I knew that and had previously passed the release forms over to the staff.

An administrator came to the desk and, somewhat embarrassed, explained that I had to wait for the police.

I couldn't quite comprehend.

'Did you say 'the police?''

'Well, yes. I'm sorry but because your mother had an accident, now that she has passed away, it becomes a police matter. They will be interviewing you before you leave the hospital. We've contacted them but we have no way of knowing when they will come.'

Aaah! Time to really gather myself: I knew I was in a very fragile state. I knew I had to drive in very busy streets for 40 minutes. I was determined not to compound the situation by having an accident so I called on my years of practising yoga.

Returning to the room where Mum still peacefully lay, I spread my shawl on the floor at the foot of the bed and lay down on my back, feet pointing away from the door, going into the 'death pose', breathing slowly and relaxing every part of my body...

Something disturbed me. When I opened my eyes I looked up to see an upside-down semi-circle of very serious young faces above police uniforms peering anxiously down at me. It was almost five a.m. Hastily righting myself I slid into a chair explaining that I didn't need any medical help - was just relaxing.

I felt so sorry for them. The youngest officers - two women and a guy - had been sent on this job and I doubted whether any of them had ever been in a room with a dead body before. They kept glancing sideways at Mum, while they very politely asked me to describe the accident.

I don't know how garbled I sounded - the event seemed so far in the past. I kept interrupting myself, trying to clear my head, trying to explain everything in consecutive order, fighting the dawning realisation that I was the only person with my mother when she fell. The police are trained to detect crime, and elder-abuse is not uncommon. My story was definitely sounding more and more crazily far-fetched and suspicious.

I desperately explained that although she was 99 all she had was dementia - she was very active and strong … she could easily drag a large, heavy wooden toolbox across the floor to a window and climb onto it. They were looking at this tiny fragile body, barely making a hump under the sheet. I could imagine their skeptical 'Really?'

Inside my head I was cringing. Heavens! Was I protesting too much? *Don't panic! Just tell the story.*

Why is it that you always feel guilty when confronted with a policeman?

I kept looking at Mum. They tried not to. When her eyes opened again (part of the rigor mortis?) I inanely said, 'Oh look! It's like she's listening!' They all looked horrified.

Notes were earnestly taken and after conferring among themselves they FINALLY gave official permission for me to be released from the ward. Somehow, I drove home safely.

∾

While I knew it had been an accident, I still felt completely responsible. After all, she was in my care. The next few days, waiting for the coroner's report, were pretty anxious for us all but relief was finally delivered. It was official - accidental death - so we proceeded with the funeral arrangements.

Out of respect for her religious beliefs, always kept private, but nevertheless very much a part of my mother, we planned the funeral in St. John's, Mona Vale, a tiny, delightful old stone church. A Bing Crosby song and an aria from The Messiah were in the music selection.

Best of all, our wonderful funeral director insisted that Banjo be included. He sat quietly next to me in the front pew and when the coffin was carried past, he slipped in behind the minister and led the congregation down the aisle to the exit. Mum would have been delighted!

A poignant touch - there had been a shortbread-making session the week before her accident, so we had the experience of eating 'Nan's shortbread' for a further couple of weeks - such a fitting legacy. She nurtured us from beyond the grave.

~

After the family departed I think I moved into a sort of limbo state, mostly staying at home but spending time at the beach every day, adjusting to the realisation of a kind of freedom I hadn't experienced for years, allowing the crowding memories to pass through my brain, just trying to rebalance myself.

My staunch friend, Lynn, fellow-carer/creative-whinger, was there on the phone every day. She was also terribly distressed. Her husband, Alan, had been moved out of their home some months before and within days of Mum's death he had begun to deteriorate. I spent a little time with her in the nursing home as she sat her vigil, waiting for the final release.

Then exactly a week after Mum's I found myself back at St. John's attending Alan's funeral.

I'd had a nasty fright during that week when I answered a knock at the door and was confronted with two more policemen, asking to come in.

They wanted a statement about the accident.

Talk about panic! *Was I under suspicion? How?* I told them we'd buried Mum - the coroner had cleared it as an accident - I'd already had a police interview the night she died. This all tumbled out as I seated them in the lounge.

They explained that the police who spoke to me were from the Crows Nest precinct, where the hospital was situated, whereas the accident had occurred in theirs so they were obliged to undertake their own investigation.

So I had to relive it again, seriously worrying whether I was giving the same facts in the same order, futilely racking my brain to remember what I'd said before, praying I wouldn't make a mistake and somehow incriminate myself!

'Well I had to lock her in at night.' A normal part of my life suddenly took on sinister overtones.

'Yes, I know she was 99 but she was very strong - she really did drag that box over to the window. She was very agile.'

I hadn't been able to eradicate the scrape marks from the verandah floor.

I ploughed on. I showed them the window - took them down onto the path where she landed. The more I talked the more bizarre it all sounded. I was visualising being hauled off to the station! But ultimately it was a formality.

They left satisfied.

I grabbed a glass of wine!

Over the next few weeks I began the slow process of taking on the grief, returning to 'normality' after years of being almost cloistered. When out somewhere in the late afternoon I'd suddenly be overcome with the panicky thought that I should be home with Mum. Or seeing an elderly lady accompanied by what I presumed to be her daughter would cause pangs of nostalgia.

One day I drove up to the Bahai House of Worship in Terry Hills, a place I'd taken Mum to a couple of times. It's such a beautiful, calming space, a nine-sided circular building, surrounded by well-tended gardens backing onto natural bushland. There is always a volunteer quietly sitting by one of the huge open doorways.

For some time I sat, contemplating, remembering, musing - absorbing the peaceful atmosphere. On leaving, as I passed the attendant I acknowledged her and she rose and enclosed me in her arms - such a beautiful, loving gesture from a complete stranger. My eyes pricking, I carried that comfort back into my life - never forgotten.

∼

It did take some effort to reintegrate, firstly staying with family and friends in Queensland and then returning to Sydney to organise the house and begin the endless sorting and distribution of a lifetime's collection, while waiting for probate.

Richard was executor and it took some time for everything to be finalised but I needed that time to adjust to being on my own once more, living in Mum's house, feeling her presence everywhere.

However, I comforted myself with the knowledge that my 'Project Mum' was complete and, on the whole, successful.

Of course there were misgivings about how I'd handled it. I had learned on the job and I'd made many mistakes but my prime aim of mostly keeping Mum happy and never letting her know she was being looked after had been achieved.

The myth - that she had lived independently until the end - had been maintained and for that I was very grateful.

Early in 2009 Richard and Soe returned to Sydney and we made the trip over to Oxford Falls. Richard watched from the car as Soe and I carried the container with Mum's ashes across the rock platforms next to the shallow creek to the cliff edge where we could look back at the tumbling waterfall.

Just as we tipped the ashes out, a strong wind-gust erupted from the gully and distributed most of them all over us!

Ah Mum! You had the last laugh!

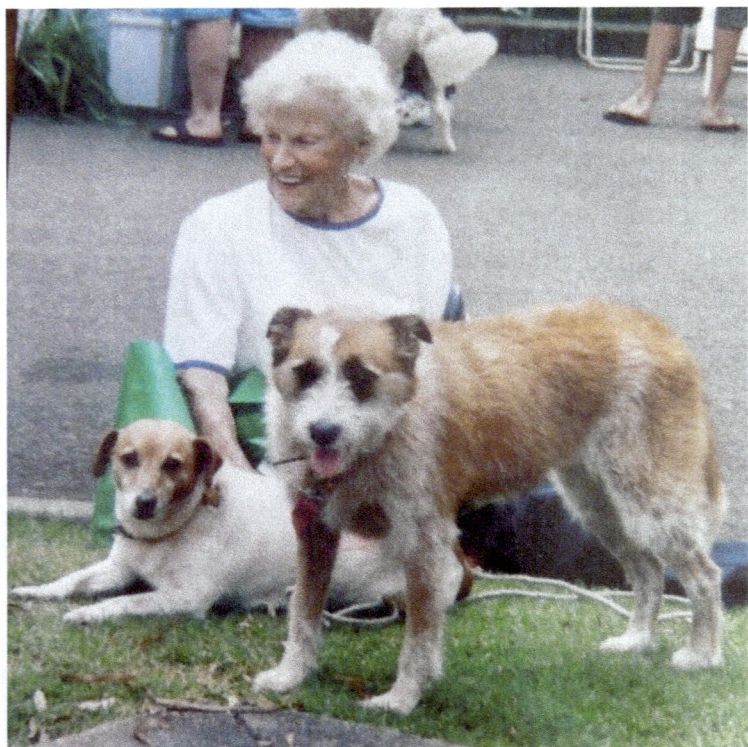

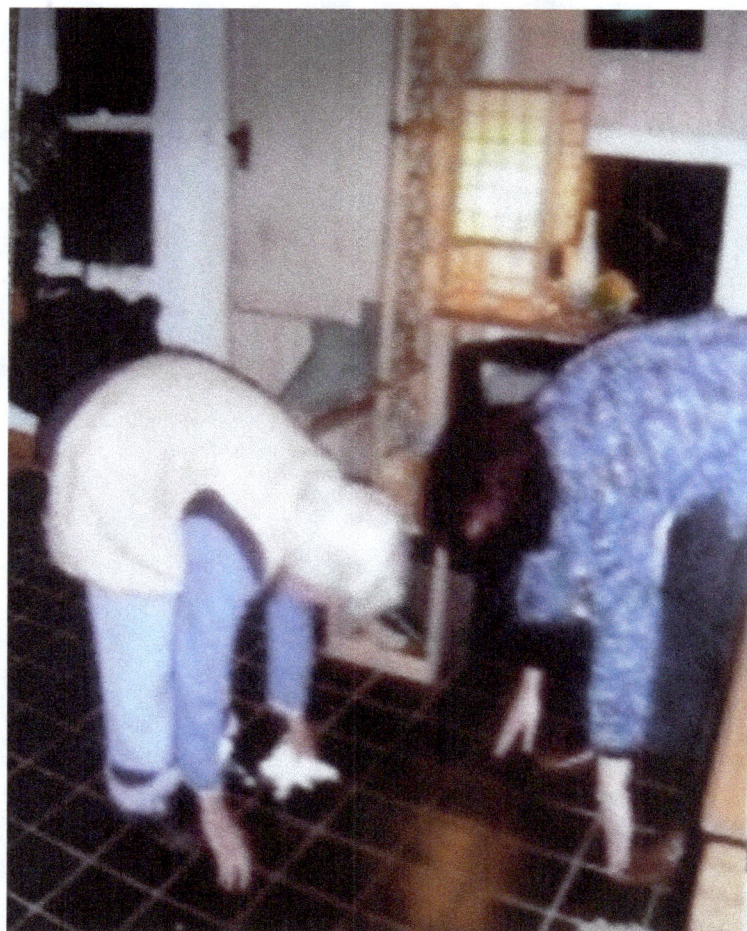

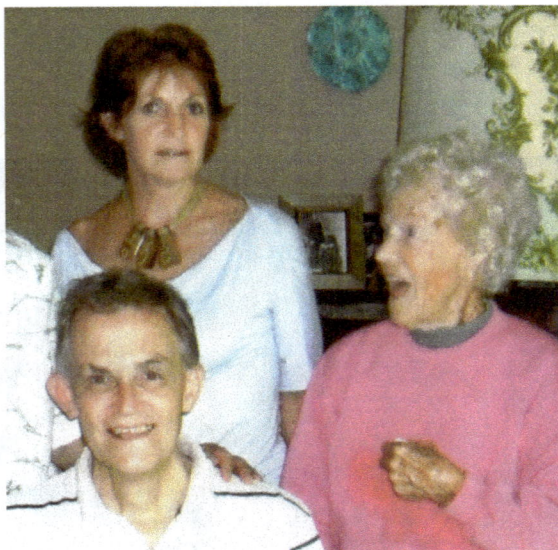

Previous pages: 1. Minding 'Podge and Banjo at a market. 2. At 99, touching her toes with Karin. Above: Mum, Richard and me. Over page: Edna's 99th birthday celebration.

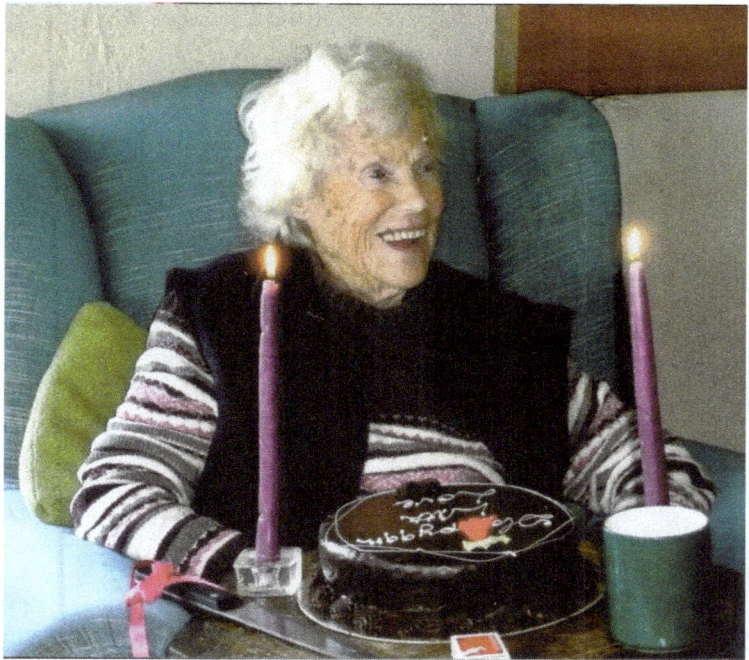

Afterword

I am ever thankful that I had the flexibility to be able to relocate to allow my mother to stay in her home right to the end. For me it was a privilege. And what a learning experience! My fascination with the phenomenal capacity of the brain continues.

My eyes still well up when I hear stories about sufferers of dementia. My actual, hands-on caring stint was relatively short - three years in all - and far less onerous than many other carers endure but I learned so much in those years and I value the experience beyond description.

My heart goes out to all who are in a caring role - so, so many loving people stalwartly soldiering on and coping, always coping.

Everyone deals with situations in their own way. I just hope they all learn to reach out for support and respite.

My message: accept, try to detach, develop strategies, then MANAGE. And ALWAYS make some time to nurture yourself.

Oh! And don't forget, when all else fails - cross your fingers!

Keep strong!

'Life is a Challenge - Meet it!
Life is a Song - Sing it!
Life is a Dream - Realise it!
Life is a Game - Play it!
Life is Love - Enjoy it!
- Bhagawan Sri Sathya Sai Baba

All quotations are from: 'A THOUSAND PATHS TO
   TRANQUILLITY' - David Baird.
   I opened this special, small book at random every morning, seeking words to help sustain me throughout the day -
just one of my tools.

Epilogue

The following year I took a wonderful trip overseas to visit Kriket and Mark in Anglesey, North West Wales, where I immersed myself in the multiple layers of history evident in the landscape, from 4000 year-old neolithic tombs to iron-age ruins. I traipsed fields to touch ancient standing stones, climbed up to a Roman fort, found the stone foundations of the ancient Welsh Kings' seat of power and wandered the ruins of Beaumaris Castle, built by Edward 1st when he conquered Wales in the 13th century.

Then I travelled to my three other long-dreamed-of destinations - places I had hardly dared hope I'd ever visit; Barcelona, to immerse myself in the architectural creations of Antoni Gaudi; Crete, to explore the phenomenal Minoan civilisation, followed by three fascinating weeks working on an archeological dig in the deserted Roman city, Sanis-era, on Menorca.

And, yes, in January, 2011, courtesy of my share of the proceeds from the sale of Mum's house I did finally buy that motorhome. It's fully self-contained and Banjo and I lived in it for over four years, joining the thousands of 'grey nomads' travelling this amazing country.

Our first extended journey of ten months was across to South Australia, up the Centre to Kathryn, then through the Kimberleys to Broome and down the West Australian Coast before heading back across the Nullabor to Queensland, taking many side trips all along the way.

By a small miracle, in 2011 Australia had experienced several years of good seasons and the entire country was green, offering wildflowers all the way and stunning photo opportunities, such as when I took a flight over Lake Eyre in full flood! When Banjo and I returned to Queensland in April, 2012, I heard that there wasn't one district on the entire continent that was drought-declared, something that hadn't happened for over twenty years and a situation that only lasted a matter of weeks.

I still travel at least 6 months of every year, commuting to new destinations, as well as visiting numerous friends and family scattered from North Queensland down through Victoria to South Australia.

Such freedom!

I call my motorhome 'Teddy', my Dad's nickname for Edna. So often I arrive somewhere and wish Mum could see it too - especially beautiful parks, gardens and wildflowers.

She travels with me.

Acknowledgments

I want to thank all my friends and family, who encouraged me to write this memoir, especially, Lynn Grierson, Beverley Harmer and Richard Hinder, who read my draft manuscript and gave me the impetus to soldier on.

Special thanks to Lynn for the 'creative whinges' - helping me though all those anguished hours when we were in our respective 'cloisters'.

Professional input from Caylie Jeffery, through the Queensland Writers' Centre and Robyn Sheahan-Bright of Justified Text really made me feel I could actually achieve a useful book and, most of all, I am eternally indebted to Edwina Shaw (edwinashaw@icloud.com) for her meticulous editing, generosity, loving enthusiasm and support. She truly got me over the line.

The sketch for my cover was kindly supplied by artist Margaret Worthington (tufdog@bigpond.com.)

Extra thanks to Mark Dawson's SPF101 course.

CARER SUPPORT

- NATIONAL DEMENTIA HELPLINE- 1800 100 500
- DEMENTIA AUSTRALIA is the national support organisation. There are head offices in each state capitol plus many regional offices. Check the website for details.
- DEPARTMENT OF SOCIAL SERVICES, *P.O. Box 9820, Canberra, A.C.T. 2601*
- CARER GATEWAY (Australian Government). Freecall 1800 422 737 www.carergateway.gov.au

AUSTRALIAN RESEARCH FACILITIES

- UNIVERSITY OF SYDNEY BRAIN AND MIND CENTRE.
- QUEENSLAND BRAIN INSTITUTE - UNIVERSITY OF QUEENSLAND.

Both of the above are undertaking important research.

- THE BRAIN CENTRE - sponsors a huge range of research, including for Alzheimers.

SUGGESTED READING

- THE FIRE INSIDE - HOW STRESS ATTACKS YOUR BODY by Caroline Williams, New Scientist magazine #3130 June 2017

- CONTENTED DEMENTIA by Oliver James, *Vermillion 2009, ISBN 9780091901813, Ebury Publishing*

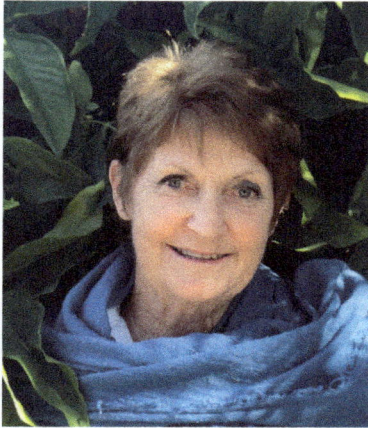

Helen Broadhurst's life has been somewhat nomadic - more by accident than design - taking her from regional N.S.W. to Sydney as a child then P.N.G. in early adulthood. There she learned various crafts from villagers, particularly traditional potting techniques in the West Sepik Province.

Returning to Australia in the mid-seventies with her family, Helen developed as a potter, teaching and conducting workshops throughout regional Queensland. During the nineties this morphed into a Community Arts place-making practice; she undertook projects making public art in many diverse communities, again travelling Queensland. Sculpture and mosaics became specialties.

Describing herself as a 'maker' rather than a writer,

throughout her different activities, she did write spasmodically for craft periodicals, as well as various professional publications.

During her time as carer for her mother, Edna, she kept notes, as well as writing copious emails and letters to her daughters, describing her mother's antics and how she dealt with their consequences.

This memoir is the result.

Please leave a review

I'd really appreciate a review of my book. My aim is to contribute to the experience of other carers.

contact: www.helenbroadhurst.com

This book is also avail as an e-book on:
    Kindle